PCOS DIET COOKBOOK FOR NEWLY DIAGNOSED

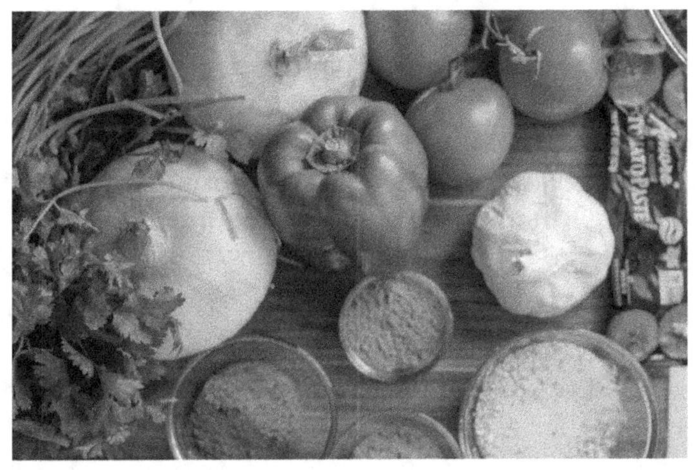

Nourishing Recipes and Lifestyle Strategies for PCOS Management and Insulin Resistance

Thelma Howard

Table of Contents

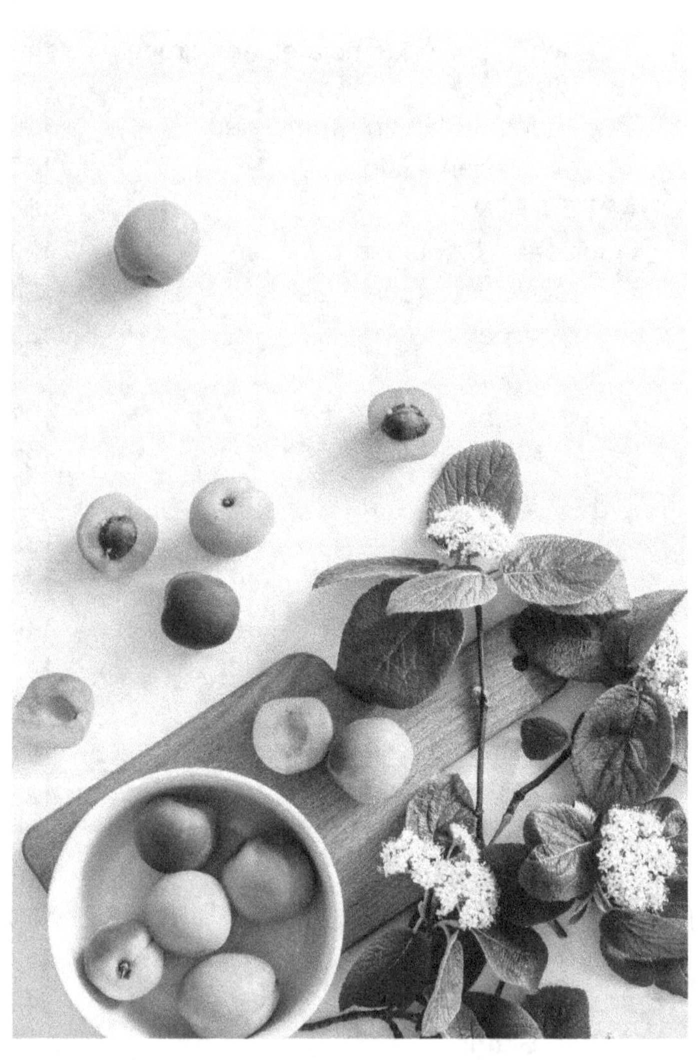

INTRODUCTION

Definition and Explanation of PCOS

PCOS, or polycystic ovarian syndrome, is a prevalent hormonal condition affecting women who are fertile. It is characterized by an imbalance of reproductive hormones, insulin resistance, and the development of multiple small cysts on the ovaries.

PCOS is a complex condition with various symptoms and manifestations, which can vary from person to person. It is estimated that around 5-10% of women of childbearing age are affected by PCOS. Although the precise origin of PCOS is unknown, a mix of environmental and genetic factors are thought to be involved.

The primary features of PCOS include:

1. **Hormonal Imbalance**: Women with PCOS have higher levels of androgens (male hormones) such as testosterone, which can disrupt the normal menstrual cycle and affect the development and release of eggs from the ovaries.

2. **Ovarian Cysts**: The ovaries of women with PCOS often contain multiple small cysts, which are fluid-filled sacs. These cysts are not harmful or

cancerous but can contribute to hormonal imbalances and interfere with normal ovulation.

3. **Menstrual Irregularities**: PCOS can cause irregular or absent menstrual periods. Some women may experience infrequent periods, while others may have heavy and prolonged menstrual bleeding.

4. **Infertility**: Due to irregular ovulation or lack of ovulation, women with PCOS may face difficulties in getting pregnant. One of the main reasons why women cannot conceive is PCOS.

5. **Other Symptoms**: PCOS is associated with a range of additional symptoms, including excessive hair growth (hirsutism) on the face, chest, and back, acne, oily skin, weight gain, insulin resistance, and metabolic abnormalities such as high cholesterol and increased risk of type 2 diabetes.

It is significant to remember that each person may experience PCOS symptoms and severity differently. Not all women with PCOS will experience every symptom, and the combination and intensity of symptoms can change over time.

The diagnosis of PCOS involves a comprehensive evaluation of a woman's medical history, physical examination, and laboratory tests. The Rotterdam criteria, which require the presence of at least two out of three criteria (oligo-ovulation or anovulation, clinical or biochemical signs of hyperandrogenism, and polycystic ovaries on ultrasound), are commonly used to diagnose PCOS.

While there is no cure for PCOS, it can be effectively managed through lifestyle modifications, including regular exercise, weight management, and a healthy diet. Medications may also be prescribed to regulate menstrual cycles, reduce androgen levels, and manage other specific symptoms.

Proper diagnosis, early intervention, and ongoing management are crucial for women with PCOS to minimize the long-term health risks associated with the condition, such as infertility, type 2 diabetes, cardiovascular disease, and mood disorders.

PCOS is a complex hormonal disorder that affects women of reproductive age. It is characterized by hormonal imbalances, ovarian cysts, menstrual irregularities, and other associated symptoms. Understanding the definition and explanation of PCOS is essential for its diagnosis, management, and addressing the unique needs of individuals affected by the condition.

PCOS Prevalence and Risk Factors

Polycystic ovary syndrome (PCOS) is a common endocrine disorder that affects women of reproductive age worldwide. Understanding the prevalence and risk factors associated with PCOS is important for identifying individuals at risk and implementing appropriate preventive measures and management strategies.

Prevalence of PCOS:

Depending on the population under study and the diagnostic criteria applied, PCOS prevalence varies. It is estimated that PCOS affects approximately 5-10% of women of childbearing age. However, the actual prevalence may be higher due to underdiagnosis and misdiagnosis. PCOS can occur in women from all ethnicities and races.

Risk Factors:

While the exact cause of PCOS is not fully understood, several risk factors have been identified that contribute to its development. These risk factors include:

1. Genetics: PCOS has a significant hereditary component. PCOS is more common in women who have a family history of the disorder. Certain genetic variations associated with insulin signaling and hormone regulation have also been linked to PCOS.

2. Insulin Resistance: One of PCOS's typical characteristics is insulin resistance. It is a condition in which the body's cells become less responsive to

the effects of insulin, leading to higher insulin levels in the blood. Insulin resistance is believed to play a significant role in the development of PCOS and its associated symptoms.

3. Obesity: Excess body weight and obesity are closely linked to PCOS. Obesity worsens insulin resistance and hormonal imbalances, increasing the risk of developing PCOS and exacerbating its symptoms. Women with PCOS are more likely to be overweight or obese compared to women without the condition.

4. Hormonal Imbalances: Elevated levels of androgens, or male hormones, such testosterone, are a hallmark of PCOS. Hormonal imbalances, including elevated androgen levels and abnormal levels of luteinizing hormone (LH) and follicle-stimulating hormone (FSH), contribute to the development and progression of PCOS.

5. Metabolic Factors: PCOS is associated with metabolic abnormalities such as dyslipidemia (abnormal lipid levels), impaired glucose tolerance, and increased risk of type 2 diabetes. These metabolic factors are thought to be interconnected with insulin resistance and hormonal imbalances in PCOS.

6. Inflammation: Chronic low-grade inflammation is believed to play a role in the development of PCOS. Inflammatory markers such as C-reactive

protein (CRP) and tumor necrosis factor-alpha (TNF-alpha) are often elevated in women with PCOS.

7. Environmental Factors: Exposure to certain environmental factors, such as endocrine-disrupting chemicals (EDCs) found in plastics, pesticides, and personal care products, may contribute to the development or worsening of PCOS symptoms. However, more research is needed to fully understand the impact of environmental factors on PCOS.

It is important to note that while these risk factors increase the likelihood of developing PCOS, not all women with these risk factors will develop the condition. PCOS is a complex disorder with a multifactorial etiology, and additional research is needed to fully elucidate its causes.

Understanding the prevalence and risk factors associated with PCOS can help healthcare professionals and individuals at risk to identify and manage the condition effectively. Early diagnosis, lifestyle modifications, and targeted interventions can help mitigate the impact of PCOS on reproductive health, metabolic health, and overall well-being.

Common Symptoms and Health Implications of PCOS

A hormonal condition known as polycystic ovarian syndrome (PCOS) affects women who are fertile. It is characterized by various symptoms, which can vary in severity and manifestation from person to person. Understanding the common symptoms and health implications of PCOS is crucial for early detection, diagnosis, and effective management of the condition.

Common Symptoms of PCOS:

1. Menstrual Irregularities: Irregular menstrual cycles are a hallmark symptom of PCOS. Women with PCOS may experience infrequent periods, prolonged periods, or completely absent periods (amenorrhea). These irregularities occur due to hormonal imbalances and disrupted ovulation.

2. Ovarian Cysts: PCOS is named after the presence of multiple small cysts on the ovaries. These cysts are not harmful but can contribute to hormonal imbalances and interfere with normal ovulation. However, it is important to note that not all women with PCOS will have visible cysts on ultrasound.

3. Hyperandrogenism: Elevated levels of androgens (male hormones) are commonly observed in women with PCOS. This can lead to symptoms such as hirsutism (excessive hair growth

on the face, chest, and back), acne, and oily skin. Hair loss or thinning of the scalp (male-pattern baldness) may also occur.

4. Weight Gain and Difficulty Losing Weight: Many women with PCOS struggle with weight management. Insulin resistance, a common feature of PCOS, can contribute to weight gain and make it challenging to lose weight. Weight gain in PCOS can further exacerbate hormonal imbalances and insulin resistance.

5. Insulin Resistance and Metabolic Abnormalities: PCOS is associated with insulin resistance, a condition in which the body's cells become less responsive to the effects of insulin. Insulin resistance can lead to elevated blood sugar levels, increased risk of type 2 diabetes, and metabolic abnormalities such as dyslipidemia (abnormal lipid levels) and high blood pressure.

6. Fertility Issues: PCOS is one of the leading causes of female infertility. Ovulation problems and irregular menstrual cycles can make it difficult for women with PCOS to conceive. However, with appropriate interventions and fertility treatments, many women with PCOS can achieve successful pregnancies.

7. Emotional and Psychological Effects: The hormonal imbalances and the impact of PCOS on fertility and body image can have emotional and

psychological implications. Women with PCOS may experience increased stress, anxiety, depression, and reduced quality of life.

Health Implications of PCOS:

1. Increased Risk of Type 2 Diabetes: Insulin resistance and metabolic abnormalities in PCOS increase the risk of developing type 2 diabetes. Regular monitoring of blood sugar levels and adopting a healthy lifestyle are essential for managing this risk.

2. Cardiovascular Disease: Women with PCOS have a higher risk of developing cardiovascular diseases such as hypertension, dyslipidemia, and heart disease. Lifestyle modifications, including regular exercise and a heart-healthy diet, are crucial for reducing this risk.

3. Endometrial Cancer: Irregular or absent menstrual periods and unopposed estrogen exposure in PCOS can lead to thickening of the uterine lining (endometrium). This increases the risk of endometrial hyperplasia and, in some cases, endometrial cancer. Gynecological examinations on a regular basis are crucial for early detection and treatment.

4. Sleep Apnea: PCOS is associated with an increased risk of obstructive sleep apnea, a condition characterized by pauses in breathing

during sleep. Sleep disturbances can further contribute to hormonal imbalances and metabolic dysregulation.

5. Psychological and Emotional Well-being: The emotional and psychological impact of PCOS should not be overlooked. The hormonal imbalances, fertility challenges, and changes in physical appearance can lead to increased stress, anxiety, depression, and decreased quality of life. Seeking support from healthcare professionals, support groups, and counseling services can be beneficial.

It is important to remember that PCOS is a heterogeneous condition, and not all women will experience the same symptoms or health implications. The severity and combination of symptoms can vary, and individualized management approaches are necessary. Early diagnosis, lifestyle modifications, and targeted interventions can help manage the symptoms and mitigate the long-term health implications associated with PCOS.

Importance of Lifestyle and Diet for PCOS Management

Polycystic ovary syndrome (PCOS) is a hormonal disorder that can significantly impact a woman's health and quality of life. While there is no cure for PCOS, adopting a healthy lifestyle and making dietary modifications can play a crucial role in managing the condition and reducing its associated symptoms. Lifestyle and diet interventions are often the first line of treatment for PCOS and can have a positive impact on hormonal balance, weight management, insulin resistance, and overall well-being.

Here are the key reasons why lifestyle and diet are important for PCOS management:

1. Weight Management: Many women with PCOS struggle with weight gain and find it difficult to lose weight. Excess weight and obesity can worsen insulin resistance and hormonal imbalances, leading to more severe PCOS symptoms. Adopting a healthy lifestyle and focusing on weight management can help improve insulin sensitivity, regulate hormone levels, and reduce the severity of PCOS symptoms.

2. Insulin Sensitivity: A typical characteristic of PCOS is insulin resistance. It is important to control insulin levels and improve insulin sensitivity to manage PCOS effectively. Regular exercise, such as aerobic activities and strength training, can help improve insulin sensitivity and glucose metabolism. Additionally, a balanced diet that includes complex carbohydrates, fiber-rich foods, and adequate protein can help stabilize blood sugar levels and reduce insulin resistance.

3. Hormonal Balance: PCOS is characterized by hormonal imbalances, including elevated levels of androgens (male hormones) and disrupted levels of luteinizing hormone (LH) and follicle-stimulating hormone (FSH). Lifestyle interventions, such as regular exercise and a healthy diet, can help regulate hormone levels and restore hormonal balance. Physical activity promotes the production of endorphins and reduces stress, which can positively impact hormone regulation.

4. Menstrual Regularity: Irregular menstrual cycles are a common symptom of PCOS. A healthy lifestyle and diet can help regulate menstrual cycles and promote ovulation. Regular exercise and weight management can improve hormone balance and increase the likelihood of regular and predictable periods.

5. Fertility Enhancement: PCOS is one of the leading causes of female infertility. Lifestyle modifications, including weight loss, regular physical activity, and a healthy diet, can improve fertility outcomes in women with PCOS. Losing even a modest amount of weight can improve ovulation and increase the chances of successful conception.

6. Cardiovascular Health: Women with PCOS are at an increased risk of developing cardiovascular diseases such as hypertension, dyslipidemia, and heart disease. Adopting a heart-healthy lifestyle,

including regular exercise, a balanced diet, and weight management, can help reduce the risk of cardiovascular problems and improve overall cardiovascular health.

7. Emotional Well-being: PCOS can have a significant impact on emotional well-being, leading to increased stress, anxiety, and depression. Regular exercise and a healthy diet have been shown to improve mood, reduce stress, and promote overall mental well-being.

When it comes to diet, there is no one-size-fits-all approach for PCOS management. However, some dietary recommendations that may be beneficial include:

- Eating a well-balanced diet full of fruits, vegetables, whole grains, lean meats, and healthy fats.
- Limiting processed foods, sugary snacks, and beverages, and refined carbohydrates.
- Including foods with a low glycemic index (GI) to help stabilize blood sugar levels.
- Incorporating fiber-rich foods to promote satiety, regulate digestion, and support weight management.
- Observing serving quantities and engaging in mindful eating.
- Considering the role of nutritional supplements, such as omega-3 fatty acids, in managing inflammation and promoting hormonal balance.

It is important for individuals with PCOS to work closely with healthcare professionals, such as registered dietitians or nutritionists, to develop personalized lifestyle and dietary plans tailored to their specific needs and goals. Regular monitoring, follow-up, and support are crucial for long-term success in managing PCOS through lifestyle and diet modifications.

In conclusion, adopting a healthy lifestyle and making dietary modifications are essential for managing PCOS effectively. Lifestyle interventions can improve weight management, insulin sensitivity, hormonal balance, menstrual regularity, fertility outcomes, cardiovascular health, and emotional well-being. Working with healthcare professionals and making sustainable changes to lifestyle and diet can significantly improve the quality of life for women with PCOS.

CHAPTER ONE

Understanding PCOS and Its Causes

Hormonal Imbalance and Insulin Resistance

Hormonal imbalance and insulin resistance are key features of several health conditions, including polycystic ovary syndrome (PCOS), type 2 diabetes, and metabolic syndrome. Understanding the mechanisms and implications of hormonal imbalance and insulin resistance is crucial for managing these conditions effectively.

Hormonal Imbalance

Hormones are chemical messengers that control a number of internal processes and activities. Hormonal imbalance refers to an abnormality in the production, secretion, or action of hormones, leading to disruptions in the body's normal physiological processes. In the context of PCOS, hormonal imbalance primarily involves the sex hormones, insulin, and other metabolic hormones.

1. Androgen Imbalance: Women with PCOS often experience elevated levels of androgens, which are male hormones such as testosterone. This

hormonal imbalance can lead to symptoms like hirsutism (excessive hair growth), acne, and male-pattern baldness.

2. Estrogen and Progesterone Imbalance: PCOS can disrupt the normal balance between estrogen and progesterone, leading to irregular or absent menstrual cycles. This imbalance can also contribute to other symptoms, such as endometrial hyperplasia and an increased risk of endometrial cancer.

3. Luteinizing Hormone (LH) and Follicle-Stimulating Hormone (FSH) Imbalance: In PCOS, there is often an elevated ratio of LH to FSH. This imbalance can disrupt the normal process of ovulation, leading to infertility and irregular menstrual cycles.

Insulin Resistance

Insulin resistance is the result of the body's cells losing their sensitivity to the pancreatic hormone insulin. Insulin plays a critical role in regulating blood sugar levels by facilitating the uptake of glucose into cells for energy production. The pancreas overproduces insulin in response to cells that grow resistant to it, which raises blood insulin levels.

1. **Causes of Insulin Resistance**: The exact causes of insulin resistance are not fully

understood but can be influenced by genetic factors, obesity, sedentary lifestyle, and dietary factors such as excessive consumption of refined carbohydrates and added sugars.

2. **Implications of Insulin Resistance**: Insulin resistance has several implications for health, including:

- Elevated Blood Sugar Levels: Insulin resistance impairs glucose uptake by cells, leading to higher levels of glucose in the bloodstream. This can eventually result in prediabetes and type 2 diabetes if left unmanaged.

- Increased Insulin Production: To overcome insulin resistance, the pancreas produces more insulin. High insulin levels can further exacerbate hormonal imbalances by increasing androgen production, disrupting ovarian function, and altering the menstrual cycle.

- Metabolic Abnormalities: Insulin resistance is often associated with metabolic abnormalities such as dyslipidemia (abnormal lipid levels), high blood pressure, and central obesity. These factors contribute to an increased risk of cardiovascular diseases like heart disease and stroke.

- Weight Gain and Difficulty Losing Weight: Insulin resistance can promote weight gain and make it challenging to lose weight. Elevated insulin levels promote fat storage and inhibit the breakdown of stored fat, leading to weight gain, particularly in the abdominal area.

- Inflammation: Insulin resistance and the subsequent high insulin levels can contribute to chronic low-grade inflammation in the body. Inflammation is associated with an increased risk of various health conditions, including cardiovascular diseases and certain types of cancer.

Managing Hormonal Imbalance and Insulin Resistance

Managing hormonal imbalance and insulin resistance is crucial for overall health and the management of conditions like PCOS and type 2 diabetes. Here are some important strategies:

1. Lifestyle Modifications: Regular exercise, such as aerobic activities and strength training, can improve insulin sensitivity, help regulate hormone levels, and assist with weight management. Adopting a healthy diet that includes whole grains, lean proteins, healthy fats, and plenty of fruits and vegetables can also support hormonal balance and improve insulin sensitivity.

2. Weight Management: Maintaining a healthy weight or losing excess weight can be beneficial for improving hormonal balance, insulin sensitivity, and overall health. A combination of regular physical

activity and a balanced diet can help achieve and maintain a healthy weight.

3. Medications: In some cases, medications may be prescribed to manage hormonal imbalances and insulin resistance. For example, in PCOS, birth control pills or other hormone-regulating medications may be used to regulate menstrual cycles and reduce androgen levels. Metformin, a medication that improves insulin sensitivity, is often prescribed for individuals with insulin resistance and type 2 diabetes.

4. Regular Monitoring and Medical Care: Regular check-ups, blood tests, and monitoring of hormone levels, blood sugar levels, and lipid profiles are important for managing hormonal imbalance and insulin resistance. This allows healthcare professionals to track progress, adjust treatment plans, and identify any potential complications.

5. Stress Management and Sleep: Chronic stress and poor sleep can contribute to hormonal imbalances and insulin resistance. Implementing stress management techniques such as mindfulness, relaxation exercises, and adequate sleepcan help reduce stress levels and improve hormonal balance.

Hormonal imbalance and insulin resistance are interconnected and play significant roles in conditions like PCOS and type 2 diabetes.

Understanding the mechanisms and implications of these imbalances is crucial for effective management. Lifestyle modifications, including regular exercise, a healthy diet, weight management, stress reduction, and adequate sleep, are key strategies for improving hormonal balance and insulin sensitivity.

Role of Genetics and Environmental Factors

The development of various health conditions is influenced by a combination of genetic and environmental factors. Both genetics and the environment play important roles in determining an individual's susceptibility to certain diseases, including chronic conditions like cardiovascular diseases, diabetes, cancer, PCOS and autoimmune disorders. Understanding the role of genetics and environmental factors is essential for comprehensively assessing PCOS and implementing appropriate preventive measures and treatment strategies.

Genetics

Genetics refers to the study of genes and their role in heredity and variation of traits in living organisms. Genes are segments of DNA that carry instructions for the development, functioning, and maintenance of the body. Genetic variations, such as mutations or polymorphisms, can influence an individual's susceptibility to certain diseases.

1. Genetic Variations: Genetic variations can influence disease risk by affecting various aspects of human biology, including metabolism, hormone regulation, immune response, and cell growth and repair. Certain genetic variations can increase the likelihood of developing specific conditions, while others may provide protection against certain diseases.

2. Genetic Disorders: Some health conditions are directly caused by genetic mutations or abnormalities. These are often inherited from one or both parents and can manifest early in life or later in adulthood. Examples of genetic disorders include cystic fibrosis, sickle cell anemia, Huntington's disease, and muscular dystrophy.

3. Polygenic Traits: Many common diseases, such as cardiovascular diseases, diabetes, and certain types of cancer, are polygenic, meaning they are influenced by multiple genetic variations. In these cases, the combined effects of several genes, each with a small impact, contribute to the overall risk of developing the disease.

4. Genetic Testing: Advances in genetic research and technology have made it possible to identify specific genetic variations associated with increased disease risk. Genetic testing can provide individuals with information about their genetic predispositions, helping them make informed

decisions about lifestyle modifications, preventive measures, and targeted treatments.

Environmental Factors

Environmental factors encompass a wide range of external influences that can impact an individual's health and disease risk. These factors include lifestyle choices, diet, physical activity, exposure to toxins, socioeconomic status, and social and cultural factors.

1. Lifestyle Factors: Lifestyle choices, such as diet, physical activity, smoking, alcohol consumption, and stress levels, can significantly influence disease risk. Unhealthy lifestyle habits, such as a sedentary lifestyle, poor diet, and tobacco use, can increase the likelihood of developing chronic diseases like heart disease, type 2 diabetes, and certain types of cancer.

2. Diet and Nutrition: Dietary choices play a crucial role in health and disease prevention. A diet high in processed foods, unhealthy fats, added sugars, and low in fruits, vegetables, whole grains, and lean proteins is associated with an increased risk of various diseases. On the other hand, a balanced and nutrient-rich diet can help reduce disease risk and promote overall health.

3. Exposure to Toxins: Environmental toxins, such as air pollution, pesticides, heavy metals, and

industrial chemicals, can have adverse effects on health. Prolonged exposure to these toxins can increase the risk of respiratory conditions, cardiovascular diseases, neurological disorders, and certain types of cancer.

4. Socioeconomic Factors: Socioeconomic factors, including income, education, occupation, and access to healthcare, can influence disease risk and health outcomes. Individuals with lower socioeconomic status often face challenges in accessing healthcare, adopting healthy lifestyle behaviors, and living in environments that support good health.

5. Social and Cultural Factors: Social and cultural factors, such as social support, community engagement, and cultural norms, can impact health behaviors and disease outcomes. Social support networks and positive social relationships have been shown to have a protective effect on health, while cultural norms can influence dietary patterns and lifestyle choices.

Interaction Between Genetics and Environment

It is important to recognize that genetics and environmental factors do not work in isolation but interact with each other to influence disease risk and outcomes. The field of epigenetics explores how environmental factors can modify gene expression and influence health outcomes. Epigenetic modifications can occur throughout a person's lifetime and can be influenced by factors such as diet, physical activity, stress, and exposure to toxins.

The interplay between genetics and the environment highlights the importance of a comprehensive approach to disease prevention and management. While genetic predispositions cannot be changed, environmental factors can be modified to reduce disease risk. Lifestyle modifications, such as adopting a healthy diet, engaging in regular physical activity, avoiding tobacco and excessive alcohol consumption, managing stress, and reducing exposure to toxins, can help mitigate genetic risks and promote better health outcomes.

Genetics and environmental factors both contribute to an individual's disease risk and health outcomes. Genetic variations can increase susceptibility to certain diseases, while environmental factors, including lifestyle choices, diet, exposure to toxins, socioeconomic status, and social and cultural factors, can further influence disease risk. Understanding the interaction between genetics and the environment is crucial for implementing effective preventive measures, personalized treatments, and lifestyle modifications to promote better health and reduce the burden of chronic diseases.

Effects of PCOS on Fertility and Reproductive Health

Polycystic ovary syndrome (PCOS) is a common hormonal disorder that affects reproductive health in women. It is characterized by several symptoms, including irregular menstrual cycles, ovarian cysts, and excessive androgen (male hormone) production. The effects of PCOS on fertility and reproductive health can be profound. Understanding the specific effects of PCOS on reproductive health is crucial for diagnosis, management, and treatment of this condition.

1. Menstrual Irregularities: PCOS often causes irregular or absent menstrual cycles due to disrupted ovulation. The process by which a developed egg is discharged from the ovary is known as ovulation. In PCOS, the hormonal imbalances, including increased levels of luteinizing hormone (LH) and decreased levels of follicle-stimulating hormone (FSH), can prevent the regular development and release of eggs. As a result, women with PCOS may experience infrequent periods, prolonged cycles, or even complete lack of menstruation (amenorrhea).

2. Ovarian Cysts: PCOS is characterized by the presence of multiple small cysts on the ovaries.

These cysts are formed when the follicles, which contain the eggs, fail to develop fully or release the eggs during ovulation. The accumulation of these fluid-filled cysts on the ovaries can disrupt normal ovarian function and contribute to hormonal imbalances.

3. Infertility: PCOS is a leading cause of infertility in women. The irregular or absent ovulation associated with PCOS can make it challenging for women to conceive naturally. Additionally, the elevated levels of androgens in PCOS can interfere with the maturation and release of eggs, further reducing fertility. Women with PCOS may require medical intervention, such as ovulation induction medications or assisted reproductive technologies like in vitro fertilization (IVF), to achieve pregnancy.

4. Increased Risk of Miscarriage: Women with PCOS have a higher risk of miscarriage compared to women without the condition. The exact reasons for this increased risk are not fully understood but may be related to hormonal imbalances, insulin resistance, and inflammation associated with PCOS. Effective management of PCOS and close monitoring during pregnancy can help minimize the risk of miscarriage.

5. Endometrial Abnormalities: PCOS can also lead to endometrial abnormalities, particularly in women who have irregular or absent menstrual cycles. The lining of the uterus, called the endometrium, may

become thicker and may not shed properly during menstruation, increasing the risk of endometrial hyperplasia (overgrowth of the endometrial tissue) and potentially leading to endometrial cancer in the long term.

6. Hormonal Imbalances: PCOS is characterized by hormonal imbalances, including increased levels of androgens (such as testosterone) and insulin resistance. These hormonal imbalances can disrupt the normal reproductive hormone feedback loop and impair the development and release of eggs. The excessive androgen production can also lead to symptoms such as hirsutism (excessive hair growth), acne, and male-pattern baldness.

7. Metabolic Abnormalities: PCOS is often associated with metabolic abnormalities, such as insulin resistance, obesity, dyslipidemia (abnormal lipid levels), and glucose intolerance. These metabolic abnormalities can further impact reproductive health and fertility. Insulin resistance, in particular, can affect the production and action of reproductive hormones, leading to hormonal imbalances and irregular ovulation.

Management and Treatment

While PCOS can have a significant impact on reproductive health and fertility, there are several management strategies and treatment options available:

1. Lifestyle Modifications: Adopting a healthy lifestyle, including regular exercise and a balanced diet, can help manage PCOS symptoms and improve reproductive health. Weight management is particularly important, as weight loss can restore ovulation and improve fertility in overweight or obese women with PCOS.

2. Medications: Various medications may be prescribed to manage PCOS-related symptoms and improve fertility. These may include oral contraceptives to regulate menstrual cycles, anti-androgen medications to reduce excessive hair growth and acne, and ovulation-inducing medications like clomiphene citrate or letrozole to stimulate egg production.

3. Assisted Reproductive Technologies (ART): For women with PCOS who struggle to conceive naturally, assisted reproductive technologies such as intrauterine insemination (IUI) or in vitro fertilization (IVF) can be effective options. These techniques can help overcome ovulation difficulties and increase the chances of successful pregnancy.

4. Management of Metabolic Abnormalities: Addressing metabolic abnormalities, such as insulin resistance and dyslipidemia, through lifestyle modifications and medications can improve reproductive health outcomes in women with PCOS. Metformin, a medication that improves

insulin sensitivity, is often prescribed to manage insulin resistance and metabolic health in PCOS.

5. Regular Monitoring: Regular medical check-ups, monitoring of menstrual cycles, hormone levels, and ultrasound evaluations can help track the progress of PCOS and assess the effectiveness oftreatment. Close monitoring during pregnancy is also important to ensure the well-being of both the mother and the baby.

PCOS can have a significant impact on reproductive health and fertility in women. The hormonal imbalances, irregular ovulation, ovarian cysts, and metabolic abnormalities associated with PCOS can make it challenging for women to conceive and maintain a healthy pregnancy. However, with appropriate management strategies, including lifestyle modifications, medications, and assisted reproductive technologies, many women with PCOS can achieve successful pregnancies.

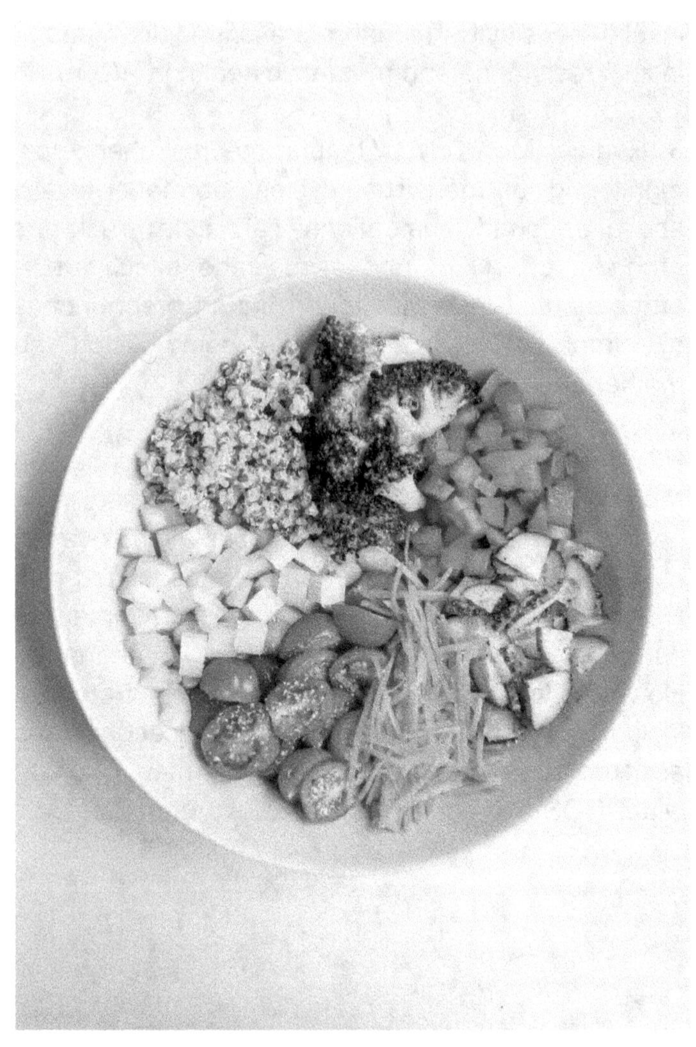

CHAPTER TWO

Understanding PCOS Diets

A PCOS-friendly diet focuses on balancing nutrient intake, stabilizing blood sugar levels, and promoting hormonal balance to manage symptoms and improve overall health outcomes. The following are key principles and guidelines for building a PCOS-friendly diet:

1. Balanced Macronutrients

Complex Carbohydrates: Choose carbohydrates that are high in fiber and low in glycemic index (GI). Examples include whole grains (brown rice, quinoa, oats), legumes (beans, lentils), fruits, and vegetables. Because they digest more slowly, these carbohydrates don't cause sudden rises in blood sugar.

Lean Proteins: Incorporate lean protein sources such as poultry, fish, tofu, tempeh, legumes, and low-fat dairy products into your meals. Protein helps promote satiety, stabilize blood sugar levels, and support muscle maintenance and repair.

Healthy Fats: Include sources of healthy fats in your diet, such as avocados, nuts, seeds, olive oil, and fatty fish (salmon, mackerel, sardines). The synthesis of hormones, mental clarity, and the uptake of fat-soluble vitamins all depend on healthy fats.

2. Managing Insulin Resistance

Limiting Refined Carbohydrates and Sugars: Minimize consumption of processed foods, sugary snacks, desserts, and beverages with added sugars. These foods can cause rapid spikes in blood sugar levels and exacerbate insulin resistance.

Balancing Meals and Snacks: Aim for balanced meals and snacks that contain a combination of carbohydrates, protein, and healthy fats. This helps slow down the absorption of glucose into the bloodstream and prevents sharp fluctuations in insulin levels.

Frequent, Small Meals: Eating smaller, more frequent meals throughout the day can help regulate blood sugar levels and prevent overeating. Incorporate snacks rich in protein and fiber to keep you feeling satisfied between meals.

3. Nutrient-Dense Foods

Colorful Fruits and Vegetables: Incorporate a variety of colorful fruits and vegetables into your diet to ensure a diverse intake of vitamins, minerals, and antioxidants. Aim to fill half of your plate with non-starchy vegetables at each meal.

Whole Grains: Choose whole grains over refined grains whenever possible. Whole grains contain fiber, vitamins, and minerals that are beneficial for overall health and can help promote satiety and weight management.

Calcium-Rich Foods: Include sources of calcium in your diet, such as low-fat dairy products, fortified plant-based milk alternatives, leafy green vegetables (kale, collard greens), and calcium-fortified foods.

4. Hydration
Water: Throughout the day, make sure you drink enough water to stay hydrated. Water is essential for cellular function, digestion, and metabolic processes. Limit intake of sugary beverages and opt for water, herbal teas, or infused water instead.

5. Mindful Eating
Portion Control: Practice portion control and mindful eating to avoid overeating and promote awareness of hunger and satiety cues.

Slow Dining: Chew your food slowly and appreciate every taste. Eating slowly can facilitate better digestion and help avoid overindulging.

A PCOS-friendly diet emphasizes whole, nutrient-dense foods while minimizing processed and sugary foods that can exacerbate insulin resistance and hormonal imbalances. By adopting a balanced approach to nutrition, individuals with PCOS can support hormone regulation, manage symptoms, and improve overall health and well-being. It's important to consult with a healthcare professional or registered dietitian to develop a personalized dietary plan tailored to individual needs and health goals.

Foods to include

Incorporating the right foods into your diet is essential for managing PCOS (Polycystic Ovary Syndrome) and promoting overall health. Here's a comprehensive guide to foods to include in a PCOS-friendly diet:

1. **Lean Proteins**
Poultry: Turkey and skinless chicken make great sources of lean protein. To reduce additional fats, choose baked, roasted, or grilling methods of preparation.

Fish: Fatty fish like salmon, mackerel, trout, and sardines provide omega-3 fatty acids, which have anti-inflammatory properties and support heart health.

Tofu and Tempeh: These plant-based protein sources are suitable alternatives for vegetarians and vegans. They are also a great source of calcium and iron.

Legumes: Beans, lentils, chickpeas, and peas are rich in protein, fiber, and complex carbohydrates. They help stabilize blood sugar levels and promote satiety.

2. Complex Carbohydrates

Whole Grains: Choose whole grains such as brown rice, quinoa, oats, barley, and whole wheat bread and pasta. Whole grains provide fiber, vitamins, and minerals, and have a lower glycemic index compared to refined grains.

Vegetables: Load up on non-starchy vegetables like leafy greens, broccoli, cauliflower, bell peppers, carrots, and Brussels sprouts. These veggies are full with vitamins, minerals, and antioxidants.

Fruits: Enjoy a variety of fruits, including berries, apples, oranges, pears, and kiwi. Opt for whole fruits rather than fruit juices to maximize fiber intake and minimize added sugars.

3. Healthy Fats

Avocado: Avocados are rich in monounsaturated fats, which are heart-healthy and help reduce inflammation. They are also a good source of fiber and potassium.

Nuts and Seeds: Almonds, walnuts, flaxseeds, chia seeds, and hemp seeds are nutrient-dense sources of healthy fats, protein, and fiber. Enjoy them as snacks or add them to salads, yogurt, or smoothies.

Olive Oil: Extra virgin olive oil is a staple of the Mediterranean diet and provides monounsaturated fats and antioxidants. Use it for dipping, dressings for salads, and cooking.

4. Dairy and Dairy Alternatives

Low-Fat Dairy: Opt for dairy products such milk, yogurt, and cheese that are either low-fat or fat-free. Calcium, vitamin D, and protein—all crucial for healthy bones—are found in dairy products.

Plant-Based Milk Alternatives: Unsweetened almond milk, soy milk, coconut milk, and oat milk are dairy-free alternatives that can be used in place of cow's milk.

5. Herbs and Spices

Turmeric: Known for its anti-inflammatory properties, turmeric can be added to curries, soups, and stir-fries.

Cinnamon: Cinnamon helps regulate blood sugar levels and adds a warm, sweet flavor to oatmeal, yogurt, and baked goods.

Ginger: Ginger has anti-inflammatory and digestive benefits. Use fresh or ground ginger in teas, marinades, and Asian-inspired dishes.

A PCOS-friendly diet emphasizes whole, nutrient-dense foods that support hormone balance, regulate blood sugar levels, and promote overall well-being. By incorporating lean proteins, complex carbohydrates, healthy fats, and a variety of fruits and vegetables into your meals, you can manage PCOS symptoms effectively and improve your quality of life. Additionally, consulting with a registered dietitian or healthcare professional can help you create a personalized nutrition plan tailored to your individual needs and goals.

Foods to Avoid

Avoiding certain foods can help manage symptoms associated with PCOS (Polycystic Ovary Syndrome) and improve overall health outcomes. Here's a comprehensive guide to foods to avoid in a PCOS-friendly diet:

1. **High Glycemic Index (GI) Foods**
Refined Grains: White bread, white rice, pasta, and baked goods made with white flour are high in refined carbohydrates and have a high glycemic index. These foods can cause rapid spikes in blood sugar levels, leading to insulin resistance and weight gain.

Sugary Snacks and Beverages: Candy, cookies, cakes, pastries, soda, fruit juices, and sweetened beverages are high in added sugars and contribute to elevated blood sugar levels and insulin resistance.

2. **Processed and Fried Foods**
Fast Food: Burgers, fries, fried chicken, and other fast food items are often high in unhealthy fats, sodium, and calories. Regular consumption of fast food can contribute to weight gain, inflammation, and metabolic disturbances.

Processed Meats: Processed meats such as bacon, sausage, hot dogs, and deli meats are high in saturated fats, sodium, and additives. They have been connected to a higher risk of heart disease as well as other illnesses.

3. **Saturated and Trans Fats**
Fatty Meats: Limit intake of fatty cuts of beef, pork, and lamb, as well as processed meats like sausage and bacon. These meats are high in saturated fats, which can contribute to inflammation and insulin resistance.

High-Fat Dairy Products: Full-fat dairy products like whole milk, cheese, and ice cream are high in saturated fats. Opt for low-fat or fat-free dairy alternatives to reduce saturated fat intake.

Trans Fats: Avoid foods containing hydrogenated or partially hydrogenated oils, which are sources of trans fats. Trans fats increase inflammation, raise LDL (bad) cholesterol levels, and are associated with an increased risk of heart disease.

4. Excessive Alcohol Consumption

Alcoholic Beverages: Limit intake of alcoholic beverages such as beer, wine, and cocktails. Alcohol contains empty calories and can contribute to weight gain and insulin resistance.

5. High-Sodium Foods

Processed and Canned Foods: Processed foods like canned soups, sauces, and snacks often contain high levels of sodium. Excessive sodium intake can lead to fluid retention, bloating, and increased blood pressure.

6. Artificial Sweeteners and Additives

Artificial Sweeteners: Avoid artificial sweeteners like aspartame, sucralose, and saccharin, which are commonly found in diet sodas, sugar-free snacks, and packaged foods. Some studies suggest that artificial sweeteners may disrupt gut microbiota and metabolism.

Food Additives: Be cautious of foods containing artificial flavors, colors, preservatives, and other additives. These additives may have negative effects on health and can contribute to inflammation and metabolic dysfunction.

By avoiding foods high in refined carbohydrates, added sugars, unhealthy fats, sodium, and artificial additives, individuals with PCOS can better manage symptoms, improve insulin sensitivity, and support overall health and well-being. Instead, focus on consuming whole, nutrient-dense foods that promote hormonal balance, regulate blood sugar levels, and reduce inflammation. Consulting with a registered dietitian or healthcare professional can provide personalized guidance and support in developing a PCOS-friendly diet plan tailored to individual needs and preferences.

CHAPTER THREE

Lifestyle Modifications for PCOS Management

Regular Exercise and Physical Activity

Regular exercise and physical activity are essential components of managing PCOS (Polycystic Ovary Syndrome) and promoting overall health and well-being. Incorporating consistent exercise into your lifestyle can help improve insulin sensitivity, regulate hormone levels, manage weight, and reduce symptoms associated with PCOS. Here's a comprehensive guide to lifestyle modifications focusing on regular exercise and physical activity for PCOS management:

1. Benefits of Exercise for PCOS

Improved Insulin Sensitivity: Exercise helps increase insulin sensitivity, allowing cells to better respond to insulin and regulate blood sugar levels. This can help reduce insulin resistance, a common characteristic of PCOS.

Hormonal Balance: Regular physical activity can help regulate hormone levels, including reducing levels of androgens (male hormones) such as testosterone, which are often elevated in individuals with PCOS.

Weight Management: Exercise contributes to weight loss and weight maintenance, which can help alleviate symptoms of PCOS, improve fertility outcomes, and reduce the risk of obesity-related complications.

Stress Reduction: Physical activity has stress-reducing effects by promoting the release of endorphins, neurotransmitters that help improve mood and reduce feelings of stress and anxiety often associated with PCOS.

Improved Cardiovascular Health: PCOS increases the risk of cardiovascular disease, but regular exercise can help improve cardiovascular health by reducing blood pressure, lowering cholesterol levels, and promoting heart function.

2. **Types of Exercise for PCOS**
Aerobic Exercise: Activities such as walking, jogging, cycling, swimming, dancing, and aerobics classes are effective forms of aerobic exercise that can improve cardiovascular fitness, burn calories, and enhance overall health.

Strength Training: Incorporating strength training exercises using resistance bands, free weights, or bodyweight exercises helps build muscle mass, increase metabolism, and improve body composition. Pay attention to complicated exercises that work several different muscle groups.

High-Intensity Interval Training (HIIT): HIIT workouts involve alternating periods of high-intensity exercise with periods of rest or lower intensity. HIIT is effective for burning calories, improving cardiovascular fitness, and boosting metabolism in a shorter amount of time.

Yoga and Pilates: Yoga and Pilates emphasize flexibility, strength, and mindfulness. These forms of exercise can help reduce stress, improve posture, enhance flexibility, and promote relaxation, all of which are beneficial for PCOS management.

3. Incorporating Exercise into Daily Life

Set Realistic Goals: Start with small, achievable goals and gradually increase the intensity, duration, and frequency of your workouts over time. Aim for at least 150 minutes of moderate-intensity aerobic exercise or 75 minutes of vigorous-intensity aerobic exercise per week, as recommended by guidelines.

Choose hobbies You Enjoy: You're more likely to persist with long-term hobbies that you enjoy. Experiment with different forms of exercise to find what suits your preferences, lifestyle, and fitness level.

Schedule Regular Workouts: Treat exercise as an important appointment and schedule it into your daily routine. Consistency is key to reaping the benefits of regular physical activity.

Be Active Throughout the Day: Incorporate physical activity into your daily life by taking the stairs instead of the elevator, parking farther away from your destination, or going for a walk during breaks at work.

4. Listen to Your Body

Pay Attention to Signs of Overexertion: Be mindful of your body's signals and avoid pushing yourself too hard, especially if you're just starting an exercise program or if you have any existing health conditions. Rest when needed and modify your workouts as necessary.

Stay Hydrated and Fuel Your Body: Drink plenty of water before, during, and after exercise to stay hydrated. Eat a balanced diet that provides adequate energy and nutrients to support your activity level and overall health.

Aerobic Exercise

Aerobic exercise, also known as cardiovascular exercise, is any activity that increases your heart rate and breathing rate while engaging large muscle groups over an extended period. It's essential for improving cardiovascular health, increasing endurance, burning calories, and reducing the risk of chronic diseases. Incorporating a variety of aerobic exercises into your fitness routine can help you stay motivated, prevent boredom, and target different muscle groups for overall fitness and health. Aim for two or more days of muscle-strengthening exercises per week in addition to at least 150 minutes of moderate-intensity aerobic activity or 75 minutes of vigorous-intensity aerobic exercise every week. Here are some examples of aerobic exercises:

1. **Walking**

Brisk Walking: Walking at a pace that elevates your heart rate and breathing, typically around 3-4 miles per hour. It's a low-impact exercise suitable for all fitness levels and can be done outdoors or on a treadmill.

2. **Running and Jogging**

Running: Moving at a faster pace than walking, running involves a continuous motion of lifting the feet off the ground and propelling forward. It's a high-impact exercise that strengthens the cardiovascular system and burns calories efficiently.

Jogging: A slower, steady-paced version of running that still elevates the heart rate and provides cardiovascular benefits. Jogging is suitable for beginners or those looking for a less intense form of aerobic exercise.

3. **Cycling**

Outdoor Cycling: Riding a bicycle outdoors is an excellent way to engage in aerobic exercise while enjoying the scenery. It's a low-impact activity that strengthens the lower body muscles and improves cardiovascular endurance.

Stationary Cycling: Using a stationary bike indoors allows you to control intensity and resistance levels while pedaling. It's convenient for home workouts and can provide an effective cardiovascular workout.

4. **Swimming**

Lap Swimming: Swimming laps in a pool is a full-body workout that engages multiple muscle groups while providing low-impact cardiovascular exercise. It's suitable for individuals of all fitness levels and can improve endurance and strength.

5. **Dancing**

Zumba: Zumba is a high-energy dance workout that combines Latin and international music with dance movements. It's a fun and dynamic way to get your heart rate up and burn calories while improving coordination and rhythm.

Aerobic Dance Classes: Aerobic dance classes, such as step aerobics or cardio dance, involve choreographed movements set to music. These classes provide a full-body workout, including cardiovascular conditioning, strength training, and flexibility exercises.

6. Group Fitness Classes

Cardio Kickboxing: Cardio kickboxing classes incorporate martial arts-inspired moves with cardio exercises to provide a high-intensity workout that improves cardiovascular fitness and coordination.

Indoor Cycling (Spinning): Indoor cycling classes involve riding stationary bikes in a group setting with motivating music and instructor-led routines. It's an intense cardiovascular workout that can be adjusted to different fitness levels.

7. Elliptical Training

Elliptical Machine: Using an elliptical machine provides a low-impact, full-body workout that simulates walking, running, or climbing stairs. It's gentle on the joints while still providing an effective cardiovascular workout.

8. Rowing

Rowing Machine: Rowing engages multiple muscle groups, including the legs, back, arms, and core, while providing a challenging cardiovascular workout. It's a low-impact exercise suitable for all fitness levels.

9. Hiking

Hiking Trails: Hiking on trails or nature paths offers a scenic way to engage in aerobic exercise while enjoying the outdoors. It challenges the cardiovascular system and strengthens leg muscles while providing mental relaxation.

10. **Jumping Rope**
Jump Rope: Jumping rope is a simple yet effective aerobic exercise that can be done almost anywhere. It improves cardiovascular fitness, coordination, and agility while burning calories quickly.

Strength and Training

Strength training exercises are essential for building muscle strength, improving bone density, boosting metabolism, and enhancing overall functional fitness. Incorporating a variety of these strength training exercises into your workout routine can help you build strength, improve muscle tone, and support overall health and fitness goals. It's essential to start with proper form, use appropriate weights, and gradually increase intensity and difficulty as you progress. Additionally, consulting with a certified personal trainer can provide personalized guidance and ensure safe and effective strength training workouts.

Here are some examples of strength training exercises targeting different muscle groups:

Upper Body
1. Push-Ups: Targeting the chest, shoulders, and triceps, push-ups are performed by starting in a

plank position with hands shoulder-width apart, lowering the body until elbows form a 90-degree angle, and then regaining the starting posture by pushing up.

2. Dumbbell Chest Press: Lie on a bench with dumbbells in hand, palms facing forward. Extend arms upward until they are straight, then lower the weights down to chest level, and press back up.

3. Dumbbell Shoulder Press: Sit or stand with dumbbells held at shoulder height, palms facing forward. Press the weights overhead until arms are fully extended, then lower back down.

4. Bent-Over Rows: Holding dumbbells, hinge at the hips while keeping the back straight. Pull the dumbbells up towards the chest, squeezing the shoulder blades together, then lower back down.

Lower Body
1. Squats: Stand with feet hip-width apart, toes pointing forward. Lower the body by bending knees and hips, keeping the chest up and the knees tracking over the toes, then push back up to standing.

2. Lunges: Step forward with one foot and lower the body until both knees form 90-degree angles. Return to standing position and repeat with the other leg.

3. Deadlifts: Stand with feet hip-width apart, holding a barbell or dumbbells in front of the thighs. Hinge at the hips while keeping the back flat, lowering the weights towards the floor, then return to standing by driving through the heels.

4. Leg Press: Using a leg press machine, sit with feet on the platform hip-width apart. Push the platform away by extending the knees, then lower it back down.

Core
1. Plank: Start in a push-up position with hands directly under shoulders and body forming a straight line from head to heels. Hold the position, engaging the core and glutes, for a specified time.

2. Russian Twists: Sit on the floor with knees bent and feet lifted off the ground. Hold a weight or medicine ball with both hands and rotate the torso from side to side, tapping the weight on the floor beside each hip.

3. Bicycle Crunches: Lie on your back with knees bent and hands behind the head. Bring one knee towards the chest while simultaneously twisting the torso to bring the opposite elbow towards the knee. Alternate sides in a pedaling motion.

4. Plank Rows: Begin in a plank position with dumbbells in hand. Pull one dumbbell up towards the chest while keeping the hips level and core

engaged, then lower the weight back down and repeat on the other side.

Full Body

1. Kettlebell Swings: Stand with feet shoulder-width apart, holding a kettlebell with both hands in front of the body. Hinge at the hips and swing the kettlebell between the legs, then explosively drive the hips forward to swing the kettlebell up to shoulder height.

2. Dumbbell Thrusters: Hold dumbbells at shoulder height with palms facing in. Perform a squat, then explosively drive through the heels to push the weights overhead, fully extending the arms.

3. Burpees: Begin in a standing position, then squat down and place hands on the floor. Jump feet back into a plank position, perform a push-up, then jump feet back towards the hands and explosively jump up into the air with arms overhead.

High-Intensity Interval Training

High-Intensity Interval Training (HIIT) involves alternating periods of intense exercise with brief recovery or rest periods. It's an efficient way to improve cardiovascular fitness, burn calories, and boost metabolism. Incorporating HIIT workouts into your fitness routine can help you maximize calorie burn, improve cardiovascular health, and increase overall fitness levels in a shorter amount of time. It's important to customize HIIT workouts to your fitness level and goals while ensuring proper form and technique to minimize the risk of injury.

Here are some examples of HIIT exercises:

1. Sprint Intervals

Outdoor Sprints: Sprint at maximum effort for 20-30 seconds, then walk or jog for 60-90 seconds to recover. Repeat for 10-15 minutes.

Treadmill Sprints: Set the treadmill to a challenging speed and sprint for 30-60 seconds, then recover with a slower pace for 60-90 seconds.

2. Bodyweight Exercises

Burpees: Perform a full-body exercise by starting in a standing position, then squat down, place hands on the ground, jump feet back into a plank position, do a push-up, jump feet back to hands, and explosively jump up into the air.

Jump Squats: Begin in a squat position, then explode upward into a jump, land softly, and immediately squat down again to repeat.

Mountain Climbers: Start in a plank position and alternate bringing knees towards the chest in a running motion while keeping the core engaged.

3. **Cardio Equipment**
Stationary Bike Sprints: Pedal at maximum intensity for 30-60 seconds, then pedal at a slower pace for 60-90 seconds to recover.

Rowing Machine Intervals: Row at high intensity for 250-500 meters, then row at a slower pace to recover for the same distance.

Elliptical Machine Sprints: Increase resistance and speed on the elliptical for 30-60 seconds, then reduce intensity for 60-90 seconds.

4. **Circuit Training**
Tabata Protocol: Perform 20 seconds of maximum effort exercise followed by 10 seconds of rest, repeated for 4 minutes (8 rounds). Exercises can include squats, push-ups, burpees, or any other high-intensity movement.

Bodyweight Circuit: Rotate through a series of bodyweight exercises (e.g., squats, lunges, push-ups, jumping jacks) with minimal rest between exercises, aiming for maximum effort during each set.

5. **Mixed Modalities**
Combination Workouts: Combine different exercises, such as jumping jacks, squat jumps, mountain climbers, and high knees, into a single HIIT workout routine, performing each exercise for a set duration followed by a short rest period.

Important Considerations

Warm-Up and Cool Down: Always begin with a dynamic warm-up to prepare the body for intense exercise and finish with a cooldown to gradually lower the heart rate and stretch muscles.

Progression: Start with shorter intervals and gradually increase the intensity, duration, and complexity of HIIT workouts as fitness levels improve.

Recovery: Allow adequate time for recovery between HIIT sessions to prevent overtraining and injury. Listen to your body and adjust intensity and frequency as needed.

Consultation: If you have any medical conditions or concerns, consult with a healthcare professional before starting a HIIT program to ensure it's safe for you.

Yoga and Pilates

Yoga and Pilates are popular mind-body exercises that focus on improving flexibility, strength, balance, and mental well-being. While they share some similarities, they also have distinct approaches and movements. Both Yoga and Pilates offer numerous physical and mental benefits, and individuals often choose based on personal preferences, fitness goals, and individual needs. Incorporating a combination of Yoga and Pilates exercises into your fitness routine can help improve overall strength, flexibility, balance, and mental clarity.

Here are examples of Yoga and Pilates exercises:

Yoga

1. Sun Salutations (Surya Namaskar): A series of flowing movements that synchronize breath with movement, typically involving forward bends, lunges, and upward and downward-facing dog poses.

2. Warrior Poses (Virabhadrasana): Warrior I, II, and III poses are standing poses that build strength and stability in the legs, while also opening the hips and chest.

3. Tree Pose (Vrksasana): Standing on one leg with the other foot placed on the inner thigh or calf, arms stretched overhead. This pose improves balance and concentration.

4. Downward-Facing Dog (Adho Mukha Svanasana): A foundational yoga pose that stretches the entire body, particularly the shoulders, hamstrings, calves, and spine, while building strength in the arms and legs.

5. Child's Pose (Balasana): A restorative pose performed by kneeling and sitting back on the heels, then folding forward with arms extended or

relaxed by the sides. It promotes relaxation and releases tension in the back and hips.

6. Corpse Pose (Savasana): A final relaxation pose performed by lying flat on the back with arms and legs extended, eyes closed, and focus on deep relaxation and conscious breathing.

Pilates

1. The Hundred: A classic Pilates exercise that involves lying on your back, lifting the head and shoulders off the mat, and pumping the arms up and down while engaging the core muscles.

2. Roll-Up: Starting lying on the back with arms extended overhead, slowly curl the spine off the mat one vertebra at a time, reaching forward towards the toes, and then rolling back down with control.

3. Single Leg Stretch: Lying on the back with knees bent, hug one knee into the chest while extending the opposite leg straight out, then switch legs in a fluid motion while maintaining abdominal engagement.

4. Plank: Similar to yoga, the plank pose is a core-strengthening exercise performed in a push-up position with the body in a straight line from head to heels, engaging the core and stabilizing muscles.

5. Pilates Bridge: Lying on the back with knees bent and feet flat on the mat, lift the hips towards the ceiling while engaging the glutes and core muscles, then lower back down with control.

6. Swan Dive: A dynamic Pilates exercise performed lying face down with arms extended overhead, lifting the chest and arms off the mat while engaging the back muscles, then lowering back down with control.

Key Differences
Yoga: Emphasizes breath control, meditation, and relaxation techniques, with a focus on holistic well-being and spiritual connection.

Pilates: Focuses on core strength, alignment, and controlled movements to improve posture, flexibility, and muscle tone, with an emphasis on functional movement patterns.

Conclusion
Regular exercise and physical activity are fundamental components of PCOS management, offering numerous physical and mental health benefits. By incorporating aerobic exercise, strength training, flexibility work, and mindful movement into your daily routine, you can improve insulin sensitivity, regulate hormone levels, manage weight, reduce stress, and enhance overall well-being. It's important to choose activities you enjoy, set realistic goals, prioritize consistency, and

listen to your body's needs. Consulting with a healthcare professional or certified fitness trainer can provide personalized guidance and support in developing an exercise program tailored to your individual needs and goals.

Stress Management Techniques

Managing stress is an important aspect of PCOS (Polycystic Ovary Syndrome) management as stress can exacerbate symptoms and disrupt hormonal balance. Incorporating stress management techniques into your lifestyle can help reduce stress levels, improve overall well-being, and alleviate the impact of PCOS on physical and mental health. Here's a comprehensive guide to stress management techniques for PCOS management:

1. **Mindfulness Meditation**
Mindfulness Meditation: Practice mindfulness meditation to cultivate present-moment awareness and reduce stress. Set aside time each day to sit quietly, focus on your breath, and observe thoughts and sensations without judgment.

Body Scan: Perform a body scan meditation by systematically bringing awareness to each part of your body, starting from the toes and moving upward to the crown of the head, noticing any areas of tension and allowing them to release.

2. **Deep Breathing Exercises**

Diaphragmatic Breathing: Practice deep breathing exercises to activate the body's relaxation response and reduce stress hormones. Inhale deeply through the nose, expanding the abdomen, and exhale slowly through the mouth, releasing tension with each breath.

Box Breathing: Try box breathing technique, inhaling for a count of four, holding the breath for a count of four, exhaling for a count of four, and holding the breath out for a count of four, repeating for several cycles.

3. **Yoga and Tai Chi**

Yoga: Engage in gentle yoga practices that focus on breath awareness, movement, and relaxation, such as Hatha yoga, Restorative yoga, or Yin yoga. Yoga can help reduce stress, improve flexibility, and promote mind-body awareness.

Tai Chi: Practice Tai Chi, a gentle martial art that combines slow, flowing movements with deep breathing and meditation. Tai Chi promotes relaxation, balance, and mindfulness while reducing stress and anxiety.

4. **Physical Activity and Exercise**

Regular Exercise: Engage in regular physical activity and exercise to reduce stress, boost mood, and improve overall health. Choose activities you enjoy, such as walking, jogging, cycling, dancing, or swimming, and aim for at least 150 minutes of moderate-intensity aerobic exercise per week.

Strength Training: Incorporate strength training exercises into your workout routine to build muscle strength, improve metabolism, and enhance body composition. Strength training can also help reduce stress and improve mood.

5. **Relaxation Techniques**
Progressive Muscle Relaxation: Practice progressive muscle relaxation by systematically tensing and releasing muscle groups throughout the body, starting from the feet and working upward to the face and scalp.

Guided Imagery: Use guided imagery or visualization techniques to create mental images of peaceful and calming scenes, such as a beach, forest, or mountain, to evoke feelings of relaxation and reduce stress.

6. **Healthy Lifestyle Habits**
Balanced Diet: Maintain a balanced and nutritious diet rich in whole foods, fruits, vegetables, lean proteins, and healthy fats to support overall health and reduce inflammation associated with stress.

Adequate Sleep: Prioritize adequate sleep and establish a consistent sleep routine to optimize rest and recovery. Aim for 7-9 hours of quality sleep per night to support hormone balance and reduce stress levels.

Time Management: Practice effective time management techniques to prioritize tasks, set realistic goals, and establish boundaries to prevent burnout and reduce stress from work and daily responsibilities.

Incorporating stress management techniques into your lifestyle is crucial for managing PCOS effectively and improving overall well-being. By practicing mindfulness meditation, deep breathing exercises, yoga, Tai Chi, regular physical activity, relaxation techniques, and adopting healthy lifestyle habits, you can reduce stress levels, balance hormones, and promote optimal health. Experiment with different stress management strategies to find what works best for you, and prioritize self-care as part of your PCOS management plan.

Adequate Sleep and Rest

Importance of Sleep: Adequate sleep is essential for hormone regulation, metabolism, immune function, and overall well-being. Poor sleep quality and insufficient sleep duration can exacerbate symptoms of PCOS, including insulin resistance, weight gain, and hormonal imbalances.

Sleep Hygiene Practices: Practice good sleep hygiene by establishing a regular sleep schedule, creating a relaxing bedtime routine, optimizing sleep environment (e.g., comfortable mattress, dark room, cool temperature), and avoiding stimulants like caffeine and electronics before bedtime.

Stress Management: Manage stress levels to promote restful sleep. Incorporate relaxation techniques such as meditation, deep breathing exercises, yoga, or mindfulness practices into your daily routine to reduce stress and improve sleep quality.

Addressing Sleep Disorders: Address any underlying sleep disorders, such as sleep apnea or insomnia, with the help of healthcare professionals. Treatment options may include lifestyle modifications, behavioral therapies, or medical interventions to improve sleep patterns and quality.

Importance of Maintaining a Healthy Weight

Impact of Weight on PCOS: Maintaining a healthy weight is crucial for managing PCOS symptoms and reducing the risk of associated health complications, including insulin resistance, type 2 diabetes, cardiovascular disease, and infertility.

Balanced Diet: Adopt a balanced and nutritious diet that focuses on whole foods, fruits, vegetables, lean proteins, and healthy fats. Limit consumption of processed foods, sugary snacks, and refined carbohydrates, which can contribute to weight gain and insulin resistance.

Regular Physical Activity: Engage in regular physical activity and exercise to support weight management, improve insulin sensitivity, and promote overall health. Together with muscle-strengthening activities, try to get at least 150 minutes a week of moderate-intensity aerobic activity or 75 minutes of vigorous-intensity aerobic exercise.

Individualized Approach: Work with healthcare professionals, registered dietitians, or certified fitness trainers to develop an individualized nutrition and exercise plan tailored to your specific needs, preferences, and health goals.

Smoking and Alcohol Cessation

Impact on PCOS: Smoking and excessive alcohol consumption can worsen symptoms of PCOS, increase the risk of infertility, exacerbate hormonal imbalances, and contribute to cardiovascular and metabolic complications.

Quitting Smoking: Quitting smoking is one of the most important steps individuals with PCOS can take to improve their health outcomes. Seek support from healthcare providers, smoking cessation programs, or support groups to develop a personalized quit plan and overcome nicotine addiction.

Reducing Alcohol Intake: Limit alcohol consumption to moderate levels or consider abstaining from alcohol altogether to reduce the risk of PCOS-related complications. Moderation is key, and individuals with PCOS should be mindful of alcohol's effects on hormone balance, liver function, and overall health.

Healthy Coping Strategies: Find healthy coping strategies and alternative activities to manage stress and emotions without relying on smoking or alcohol. Explore hobbies, social activities, exercise, and relaxation techniques as healthier ways to cope with stress and unwind.

Lifestyle modifications are key components of managing PCOS (Polycystic Ovary Syndrome) effectively and improving overall health outcomes. Adequate sleep and rest, maintaining a healthy weight, and cessation of smoking and alcohol consumption are critical aspects of lifestyle changes for individuals with PCOS. By prioritizing sleep hygiene, adopting a balanced diet, engaging in regular physical activity, and quitting smoking and reducing alcohol intake, individuals with PCOS can improve hormonal balance, promote weight management, and reduce the risk of associated health complications.

CHAPTER FOUR

Breakfast Recipes

Here are delicious and easy-to-prepare breakfast recipes tailored for individuals with PCOS, focusing on high-protein, low-carb options to support insulin resistance:

Veggie and Egg Breakfast Bowl

Ingredients
- 2 large eggs
- Half a cup of chopped bell peppers, any color
- 1/4 cup diced onion
- 1/4 cup diced tomatoes
- 1 cup fresh spinach
- 1 tablespoon olive oil
- Salt and pepper to taste
- Optional toppings: avocado slices, salsa, shredded cheese

Method
1. Heat olive oil in a skillet over medium heat. Add diced bell peppers and onions and sauté until softened, about 3-4 minutes.
2. Add diced tomatoes and fresh spinach to the skillet. Cook until spinach is wilted and tomatoes are softened, about 2 minutes.
3. Push the vegetables to one side of the skillet and crack two eggs into the empty space. Cook the

eggs sunny-side up or scrambled to your preferred consistency.

4. Season the eggs and vegetables with salt and pepper to taste.

5. Serve the eggs and vegetables in a bowl, topped with optional avocado slices, salsa, or shredded cheese if desired.

Greek Yogurt Parfait

Ingredients

- 1/2 cup plain Greek yogurt
- 1/4 cup fresh berries (such as strawberries, blueberries, or raspberries)
- 1 tablespoon chopped nuts (such as almonds, walnuts, or pecans)
- 1 tablespoon chia seeds
- 1/4 teaspoon cinnamon
- Taste-tested optional sweetener (like stevia or honey).

Method

1. In a small bowl or glass, layer half of the Greek yogurt.

2. Add half of the fresh berries on top of the yogurt layer.

3. Sprinkle half of the chopped nuts and chia seeds over the berries.

4. Sprinkle a pinch of cinnamon over the nuts and seeds.

5. Repeat the layers with the remaining Greek yogurt, berries, nuts, chia seeds, and cinnamon.

6. Drizzle optional sweetener over the top if desired.

7. Serve immediately or refrigerate until ready to eat.

Spinach and Feta Egg Muffins

Ingredients:
- 6 large eggs
- 1 cup fresh spinach, chopped
- 1/2 cup feta cheese, crumbled
- 1/4 cup red bell pepper, diced
- 1/4 cup onion, diced
- 1/4 teaspoon garlic powder
- Salt and pepper to taste
- Cooking spray or olive oil for greasing

Preparation
1. Preheat your oven to 350°F (175°C).

2. Using a whisk, beat the eggs thoroughly in a mixing bowl.

3. Add the chopped spinach, feta cheese, red bell pepper, onion, garlic powder, salt, and pepper to the bowl. Mix well to combine.

4. Grease a muffin tin with cooking spray or lightly coat with olive oil.

5. Pour the egg mixture evenly into the muffin cups, filling each one about three-quarters full.

6. Bake in the preheated oven for 20-25 minutes or until the egg muffins are set and slightly golden on top.

7. Remove from the oven and let them cool for a few minutes before removing them from the muffin tin.

8. Serve warm or refrigerate for later use. These egg muffins can be stored in an airtight container in the refrigerator for up to 4 days.

Berry and Almond Smoothie Bowl

Ingredients:
- 1/2 cup frozen mixed berries (such as strawberries, blueberries, raspberries)
- 1/2 ripe banana, sliced and frozen
- 1/2 cup plain Greek yogurt
- 1/4 cup almond milk (or any other type of milk)
- 2 tablespoons almond butter
- 1 tablespoon chia seeds (optional)
- One tablespoon of optionally sweetened maple syrup or honey.
- Toppings: Fresh berries, sliced almonds, granola, shredded coconut

Method:
1. In a blender, combine the frozen berries, frozen banana slices, Greek yogurt, almond milk, almond butter, chia seeds, and honey or maple syrup (if using).

2. Blend on high speed until smooth and creamy, adding more almond milk if needed to reach your desired consistency.

3. Pour the smoothie into a bowl.

4. Top the smoothie bowl with fresh berries, sliced almonds, granola, and shredded coconut for added texture and flavor.

5. Serve immediately and enjoy with a spoon.

Spinach and Mushroom Frittata

Ingredients:
  - 2 eggs
  - 1/4 cup of water
  - 1 cup of fresh spinach
  - 1/2 cup of sliced mushrooms
  - Salt and pepper to taste
  - 1/4 cup of shredded cheese (optional)

Method:
  1. Set the oven's temperature to 175°C/350°F.
  2. In a bowl, whisk together the eggs and water.
  3. Add the fresh spinach and sliced mushrooms to the egg mixture.
  4. Pour the mixture into a greased oven-safe pan.
  5. Season with salt and pepper.
  6. Sprinkle shredded cheese on top if desired.
  7. Bake for 15-20 minutes or until the frittata is set and the edges are golden brown.
  8. Cut into slices and serve.

This frittata is a nutritious and balanced breakfast option for individuals with PCOS, providing protein and healthy fats to support balanced blood sugar levels.

Oatmeal's breakfast recipes for PCOS patients

5 delicious and easy-to-prepare oatmeal breakfast recipes for PCOS patients:

1. Basic Oatmeal
Ingredients:
- 1/2 cup of steel-cut oats,
- one cup of almond milk without sugar.
- 1 tablespoon of chia seeds, sweetener of your choice (optional).

Method:
Cook the oats with almond milk, add chia seeds and sweetener, if desired. Serve warm.

2. PCOS-Friendly Oatmeal
Ingredients:
- 1/2 cup of steel-cut oats
- 1 cup of unsweetened almond milk
- 1 tablespoon of almond meal
- 1 tablespoon of cashew nuts
- 1 tablespoon of shredded coconut
- 1 tablespoon of flaxseed/linseed meal
- Half a teaspoon of cinnamon powder from Ceylon.

Method:
Cook the oats with almond milk, add the remaining ingredients, and serve warm.

3. Overnight Oats

Ingredients:
- 1/2 cup of steel-cut oats
- Half a cup of almond milk without sugar
- 1 tablespoon of chia seeds
- 1 tablespoon of chunky peanut butter
- 1/2 cup of fresh or frozen strawberries.

Method:

Mix the oats, almond milk, chia seeds, and peanut butter in a jar or glass. Add strawberries and refrigerate overnight. Serve cold or warm.

4. Oatmeal with Berries and Nuts

Ingredients:
- 1/2 cup of steel-cut oats
- one cup of almond milk without sugar
- 1/2 cup of mixed berries, 1 tablespoon of chopped nuts.

Method:

Cook the oats with almond milk, add berries and nuts, and serve warm.

5. Oatmeal with Cinnamon and Fruit

Ingredients:
- 1/2 cup of steel-cut oats
- 1 cup of unsweetened almond milk
- 1/2 teaspoon of ground Ceylon cinnamon
- 1/2 cup of sliced fruit (e.g., banana, apple).

Method:

Cook the oats with almond milk, add cinnamon and fruit, and serve warm.

These oatmeal recipes are designed to provide a balance of protein, healthy fats, and low glycemic index carbs, which are beneficial for individuals with PCOS.

Chia Pudding

Ingredients:
- 1/4 cup chia seeds
- One cup of unsweetened almond milk, or any other type of milk you prefer
- One tablespoon (optional, for sweetness) of honey or maple syrup
- 1/2 teaspoon vanilla extract
- Fresh berries or sliced fruits for topping (optional)

Method:
1. In a mixing bowl or jar, combine the chia seeds, unsweetened almond milk, honey or maple syrup (if using), and vanilla extract.
2. Stir the mixture well to ensure the chia seeds are evenly distributed and not clumped together.
3. Cover the bowl or jar and refrigerate for at least 4 hours or overnight to allow the chia seeds to absorb the liquid and thicken into a pudding-like consistency.
4. After refrigeration, give the chia pudding a good stir to break up any clumps and ensure a smooth texture.
5. Serve the chia pudding in individual bowls or jars.

6. Top each serving with fresh berries or sliced fruits for added flavor, texture, and nutritional benefits.

7. Enjoy your delicious and nutritious chia pudding breakfast!

Time Duration:
- Preparation Time: 5 minutes
- Refrigeration Time: At least 4 hours or overnight

- Adjust the sweetness of the chia pudding by adding more or less honey or maple syrup according to your taste preferences.

- Feel free to customize your chia pudding with various toppings such as nuts, seeds, shredded coconut, or cocoa nibs for added crunch and flavor.

- Chia pudding can be made in advance and stored in the refrigerator for up to 3-4 days, making it a convenient and healthy breakfast option for busy mornings.

- Experiment with different flavors by adding cocoa powder, cinnamon, or almond extract to the chia pudding mixture for variety.

Chia pudding is a versatile and nutritious breakfast option that can help support hormone balance and blood sugar control in individuals with PCOS. Enjoy this delicious and satisfying dish as part of your PCOS management routine.

PCOS-Friendly Waffles

Ingredients:

- 1 cup almond flour
- 2 tablespoons coconut flour
- 1 teaspoon baking powder
- 1/4 teaspoon salt
- 2 large eggs
- 1/4 cup almond milk, unsweetened (or any other type of milk)
- 2 tablespoons melted coconut oil (or melted butter)
- One tablespoon of optionally sweetened maple syrup or honey
- 1 teaspoon vanilla extract

Method:
1. Combine the almond flour, coconut flour, baking powder, and salt in a mixing dish.
2. In another bowl, beat the eggs, then add almond milk, melted coconut oil, honey or maple syrup (if using), and vanilla extract. Mix until well combined.
3. Gradually add the wet ingredients to the dry ingredients, stirring until a smooth batter forms. Allow batter to sit for five minutes to thicken.
4. Preheat your waffle iron according to the manufacturer's instructions.
5. Lightly grease the waffle iron with coconut oil or cooking spray.
6. After pouring the batter onto the heated waffle iron, fry it as directed by the maker, until it turns golden and crispy.
7. Repeat with the remaining batter.

8. Serve the waffles warm with your favorite toppings, such as fresh berries, Greek yogurt, or a drizzle of honey or maple syrup.

Time Duration:
- Preparation Time: 10 minutes
- Cooking Time: 5-7 minutes per batch

PCOS-Friendly Pancakes:

Ingredients:
- 1 cup almond flour
- 2 tablespoons coconut flour
- 1 teaspoon baking powder
- 1/4 teaspoon salt
- 2 large eggs
- 1/4 cup almond milk, unsweetened (or any other type of milk)
- 2 tablespoons melted coconut oil (or melted butter)
- One tablespoon of optionally sweetened maple syrup or honey
- 1 teaspoon vanilla extract

Method:
1. Combine the almond flour, coconut flour, baking powder, and salt in a mixing dish.
2. In another bowl, beat the eggs, then add almond milk, melted coconut oil, honey or maple syrup (if using), and vanilla extract. Mix until well combined.
3. Gradually add the wet ingredients to the dry ingredients, stirring until a smooth batter forms.

4. Grease a non-stick skillet or griddle with cooking spray or coconut oil and heat it over medium heat.
5. Pour about 1/4 cup of batter onto the skillet for each pancake.
6. Cook until bubbles form on the surface of the pancake and the edges look set, about 2-3 minutes. Brown for an additional one to two minutes after flipping.
7. Repeat with the remaining batter.
8. Serve the pancakes warm with your favorite toppings, such as sliced bananas, chopped nuts, or a dollop of Greek yogurt.

Time Duration:
- Preparation Time: 10 minutes
- Cooking Time: 5-6 minutes per batch

PCOS-Friendly Crepes:

Ingredients:
- 1 cup almond flour
- 2 large eggs
- 1/2 cup almond milk, unsweetened (or any other type of milk)
- 1 tablespoon melted coconut oil (or melted butter)
- One tablespoon of optionally sweetened maple syrup or honey
- 1 teaspoon vanilla extract
- Pinch of salt

Method:
1. In a mixing bowl, whisk together almond flour, eggs, almond milk, melted coconut oil, honey or maple syrup (if using), vanilla extract, and a pinch of salt until smooth.
2. Over medium heat, preheat a nonstick skillet or crepe pan.
3. Lightly grease the skillet with coconut oil or cooking spray.
4. Pour about 1/4 cup of batter onto the skillet and swirl to spread the batter thinly and evenly.
5. Cook for 1-2 minutes until the edges of the crepe start to lift and the bottom is golden brown.
6. Carefully flip the crepe and cook for another 1-2 minutes until cooked through.
7. Repeat with the remaining batter, stacking the cooked crepes on a plate.
8. Serve the crepes warm with your favorite fillings, such as Greek yogurt, fresh fruit, nut butter, or a drizzle of honey or maple syrup.

Time Duration:
- Preparation Time: 10 minutes
- Cooking Time: 2-3 minutes per crepe

- Waffle, Pancake and Crepes recipes use almond flour and coconut flour instead of refined wheat flour, making them lower in carbohydrates and higher in fiber, which can help stabilize blood sugar levels.

- Customize your waffles, pancakes, and crepes with your favorite toppings and fillings to suit your taste preferences.
- These breakfast options can be made in advance and stored in the refrigerator or freezer for quick and easy meals during busy mornings.

Breakfast Burritos

Ingredients:
- 4 large eggs
- One tablespoon of coconut oil or olive oil
- Half a cup of chopped bell peppers, any color
- 1/2 cup diced onions
- 1 cup spinach, chopped
- 1/2 teaspoon garlic powder
- Salt and pepper to taste
- 4 whole wheat or low-carb tortillas
- Half a cup of shredded cheese, such mozzarella or cheddar
- Optional toppings: salsa, avocado slices, Greek yogurt

Method:
1. In a bowl, whisk together the eggs until well beaten. Add pepper, salt, and garlic powder for seasoning.
2. Heat olive oil or coconut oil in a skillet over medium heat.
3. Add diced bell peppers and onions to the skillet and sauté until softened, about 3-4 minutes.

4. Add chopped spinach to the skillet and cook until wilted, about 1-2 minutes.

5. Push the vegetables to one side of the skillet and pour the beaten eggs into the empty space.

6. Scramble the eggs until cooked through, stirring occasionally to combine with the vegetables.

7. Warm the tortillas in a separate skillet or microwave for a few seconds until pliable.

8. Divide the scrambled eggs and vegetable mixture evenly among the tortillas.

9. Sprinkle shredded cheese over the eggs in each tortilla.

10. Add optional toppings such as salsa, avocado slices, or Greek yogurt if desired.

11. Roll up the tortillas tightly to form burritos.

12. Serve the breakfast burritos immediately or wrap them in foil for a convenient grab-and-go meal.

Time Duration:
- Preparation Time: 10 minutes
- Cooking Time: 10 minutes

- You can customize your breakfast burritos by adding ingredients like cooked turkey or chicken sausage, black beans, diced tomatoes, or sliced mushrooms.

- Choose whole wheat or low-carb tortillas to keep the carbohydrate content lower and provide more fiber and nutrients.

- Make a batch of breakfast burritos ahead of time and store them in the refrigerator or freezer for quick and convenient breakfast options during busy mornings.

- Feel free to experiment with different herbs and spices to enhance the flavor of your breakfast burritos, such as paprika, cumin, or chili powder.

Enjoy these PCOS-friendly breakfast burritos as a satisfying and nutritious way to start your day.

Avocado and Egg Toast:

Ingredients:
- 1 ripe avocado
- 2 slices whole grain bread (choose low-carb bread for a lower glycemic index option)
- 2 eggs
- Salt and pepper to taste
- Optional toppings: sliced tomatoes, microgreens, red pepper flakes, or feta cheese

Method:
1. Slice the avocado in half, remove the pit, and scoop the flesh into a small bowl. Using a fork, mash the avocado until it's smooth.
2. Toast the whole grain bread slices until golden brown and crispy.
3. While the bread is toasting, heat a non-stick skillet over medium heat. Crack the eggs into the skillet and cook them to your desired level of doneness (fried, scrambled, or poached). Season with salt and pepper.
4. Spread the mashed avocado evenly onto the toasted bread slices.

5. Top each avocado toast with a cooked egg.
6. Add optional toppings such as sliced tomatoes, microgreens, red pepper flakes, or feta cheese for extra flavor and nutrition.
7. Serve the avocado and egg toast immediately while warm.

Time Duration:
- Preparation Time: 5 minutes
- Cooking Time: 5 minutes

- Choose whole grain bread for added fiber and nutrients, which can help stabilize blood sugar levels.
- Avocado provides healthy fats and fiber, while eggs offer high-quality protein, making this breakfast option satisfying and nutritious.
- Experiment with different toppings and seasonings to suit your taste preferences and add variety to your breakfast routine.
- You can also add a squeeze of lemon juice or a drizzle of hot sauce for extra flavor.
- Enjoy this avocado and egg toast alongside a serving of fresh fruit or a small handful of nuts for a balanced and satisfying meal.
This quick and easy avocado and egg toast is a nutritious breakfast option for PCOS patients, providing essential nutrients and supporting hormonal balance.

Coconut Flour Pancakes:

Ingredients:
- 1/2 cup coconut flour
- 4 eggs
- 1/2 cup unsweetened almond milk (or any dairy-free milk alternative)
- 2 tablespoons coconut oil, melted
- One tablespoon of optionally sweetened maple syrup or honey
- 1 teaspoon vanilla extract
- 1/2 teaspoon baking powder
- Pinch of salt
- Use cooking spray or coconut oil to coat the skillet.

Method:
1. In a mixing bowl, whisk together the eggs, almond milk, melted coconut oil, honey or maple syrup (if using), and vanilla extract until well combined.
2. In a separate bowl, sift together the coconut flour, baking powder, and salt.
3. Stirring constantly, gradually incorporate the dry ingredients into the wet components until a smooth batter develops. To thicken, let the batter sit for a few minutes.
4. Lightly coat a non-stick skillet or griddle with cooking spray or coconut oil before heating it to medium heat.

5. Pour about 1/4 cup of batter onto the skillet for each pancake, spreading it out slightly with the back of a spoon.
6. Cook the pancakes for 2-3 minutes, or until bubbles form on the surface and the edges look set.
7. Carefully flip the pancakes and cook for another 1-2 minutes until golden brown and cooked through.
8. Repeat with the remaining batter, adding more coconut oil or cooking spray to the skillet as needed.
9. Serve the pancakes warm with your favorite toppings, such as fresh berries, sliced bananas, or a drizzle of honey or maple syrup.

Time Duration:
- Preparation Time: 10 minutes
- Cooking Time: 10 minutes

- Coconut flour is naturally gluten-free and high in fiber, making it a great option for individuals with PCOS.
- Adjust the sweetness of the pancakes by adding more or less honey or maple syrup according to your taste preferences.
- You can customize your pancakes by adding ingredients like cinnamon, nutmeg, or shredded coconut to the batter for extra flavor.
- Serve the pancakes with dairy-free yogurt, nut butter, or a sprinkle of nuts and seeds for added protein and healthy fats.

- Leftover pancakes can be stored in an airtight container in the refrigerator for up to 3 days or frozen for longer storage. Reheat in the toaster or microwave before serving.

These coconut flour pancakes are delicious, gluten-free, and dairy-free, making them a satisfying and nutritious breakfast option for individuals with PCOS. Enjoy them as part of a balanced meal to support your health and well-being.

General Tips

- These breakfast recipes can be customized based on personal preferences and dietary restrictions. You are welcome to change or add items to suit your taste.

- Recipes are rich in protein, low in carbohydrates, gluten-free and dairy-free, and packed with nutrients to support insulin resistance and overall health for individuals with PCOS.

- Experiment with different vegetables, fruits, nuts, and seeds to create variety in your breakfast routine while still prioritizing high-protein, low-carb options etc.

Enjoy these nutritious and satisfying breakfast options to kickstart your day with energy and balance, supporting your PCOS management goals.

CHAPTER FIVE

Lunch Recipes

Here are lunch recipes that are quick, easy, and suitable for individuals with PCOS. These recipes emphasize the use of whole grains, lean proteins, and healthy fats. Additionally, I've included options for both vegetarian and vegan diets:

Quinoa Salad with Roasted Vegetables

Ingredients:
- 1 cup cooked quinoa
- Assorted roasted vegetables (such as bell peppers, zucchini, eggplant, and cherry tomatoes)
- 2 tablespoons extra virgin olive oil
- Juice of 1 lemon
- Salt and pepper to taste
- Optional: crumbled feta cheese or toasted nuts for added flavor and texture

Preparation:
1. As directed on the package, prepare the quinoa and allow it to cool.
2. Preheat the oven to 400°F (200°C). After tossing the vegetables with salt, pepper, and olive oil, roast them until soft.
3. In a large bowl, combine the cooked quinoa, roasted vegetables, lemon juice, and additional toppings if desired. Mix well.

4. Adjust the seasoning to taste and serve at room temperature or chilled.

Chickpea Salad Wrap

Ingredients:
- 1 can chickpeas, drained and rinsed
- 1/4 cup diced cucumber
- 1/4 cup diced tomatoes
- 2 tablespoons finely chopped red onion
- 2 tablespoons chopped fresh parsley
- Juice of 1 lemon
- 2 tablespoons extra virgin olive oil
- Salt and pepper to taste
- Whole grain wraps or lettuce leaves for serving

Preparation:
1. In a bowl, mash the chickpeas with a fork or potato masher until they are partially mashed.
2. Add the cucumber, tomatoes, red onion, parsley, lemon juice, olive oil, salt, and pepper. Mix well to combine.
3. As needed, taste and adjust the seasoning.
4. Warm the whole grain wraps or use lettuce leaves as a wrap. Spoon the chickpea salad onto the wrap and roll it up.
5. Serve immediately or pack it for a convenient on-the-go lunch.

Lentil and Vegetable Stir-Fry

Ingredients:
- 1 cup cooked lentils

- Assorted stir-fry vegetables (such as bell peppers, broccoli, snap peas, and carrots)
- 2 tablespoons low-sodium soy sauce or tamari (gluten-free option)
- 1 tablespoon sesame oil
- 2 cloves garlic, minced
- 1 teaspoon grated fresh ginger
- Crushed red pepper flakes (optional)
- Cooked brown rice or quinoa for serving

Preparation:

1. Heat the sesame oil in a big skillet or wok over medium-high heat.
2. Include the optional red pepper flakes, grated ginger, and chopped garlic. Stir-fry until aromatic, about 30 seconds.
3. Add the vegetables to the skillet and stir-fry until they are tender-crisp, about 4-5 minutes.
4. Add the cooked lentils and soy sauce/tamari to the skillet. Stir-fry for two to three more minutes to thoroughly heat all the ingredients.
5. Serve the lentil and vegetable stir-fry over cooked brown rice or quinoa.

Caprese Salad with Grilled Tofu

Ingredients:
- One solid tofu block, drained and compressed
- 1 cup cherry tomatoes, halved
- 1 cup fresh basil leaves
- 4 ounces fresh mozzarella cheese (or vegan mozzarella alternative), sliced

- 2 tablespoons extra virgin olive oil
- Balsamic vinegar or balsamic glaze for drizzling
- Salt and pepper to taste

Preparation:
1. Turn on the medium heat and preheat a grill or grill pan. Slice the tofu, then grill it until it gets a light brown color on both sides.
2. In a large bowl, combine the cherry tomatoes, basil leaves, and mozzarella cheese.
3. Sprinkle salt and pepper on top of the salad and drizzle with olive oil. Gently toss to mix.
4. Arrange the grilled tofu slices on a plate and top with the caprese salad mixture.
5. Drizzle with balsamic vinegar or balsamic glaze and serve.

Zucchini Noodles with Pesto

Ingredients:
- 2 medium zucchinis, spiralized or thinly sliced
- 1/4 cup of ready-made or store-bought pesto
- Cherry tomatoes, halved
- Toasted pine nuts for garnish
- Salt and pepper to taste

Preparation:
1. In a large skillet, heat a small amount of olive oil over medium heat.
2. Add the zucchini noodles and cook for 2-3 minutes until they are tender but still slightly crisp.

3. Stir in the pesto and cherry tomatoes, and cook for an additional 1-2 minutes until heated through.
4. To taste, add salt and pepper for seasoning.
5. Transfer the zucchini noodles to a serving plate and garnish with toasted pine nuts.

Black Bean and Quinoa Stuffed Bell Peppers (Vegetarian)

Ingredients:
- 4 bell peppers, any color
- 1 cup cooked quinoa
- 1 can black beans, drained and rinsed
- 1/2 cup corn kernels
- 1/2 cup diced tomatoes
- 1/4 cup diced red onion
- 1/4 cup chopped fresh cilantro
- 1 teaspoon cumin
- 1/2 teaspoon chili powder
- Salt and pepper to taste
- Optional toppings: shredded cheese, avocado slices, sour cream (use vegan alternatives if desired)

Preparation:
1. Preheat the oven to 375°F (190°C). Remove the seeds and membranes from the bell peppers by cutting off the tops.
2. In a large bowl, combine the cooked quinoa, black beans, corn kernels, diced tomatoes, red onion, cilantro, cumin, chili powder, salt, and pepper. Mix well.

3. Spoon the quinoa and black bean mixture into the hollowed-out bell peppers.
4. Place the stuffed bell peppers in a baking dish and cover with foil.
5. Bake the peppers for 25 to 30 minutes, or until they are soft.
6. Remove from the oven and let them cool for a few minutes before serving.
7. Top with optional toppings if desired and enjoy.

Chickpea and Vegetable Curry (Vegan)

Ingredients:
- 1 can chickpeas, drained and rinsed
- 1 cup diced vegetables (such as bell peppers, carrots, zucchini, and cauliflower)
- 1 can coconut milk
- 1 tablespoon curry powder
- 1 teaspoon ground cumin
- 1/2 teaspoon ground turmeric
- 1/4 tsp cayenne (adjust according to taste)
- Salt to taste
- Fresh cilantro for garnish
- Cooked brown rice or quinoa for serving

Preparation:
1. In a large skillet or pot, heat a small amount of oil over medium heat.
2. Add the diced vegetables and sauté until they are slightly softened.

3. Stir in the curry powder, cumin, turmeric, and cayenne pepper. Cook for 1-2 minutes until fragrant.

4. Add the chickpeas and coconut milk to the skillet. Stir well to combine.

5. Simmer for 10-15 minutes, or until the vegetables are tender and the flavors are well combined.

6. Season with salt to taste.

7. Serve the chickpea and vegetable curry over cooked brown rice or quinoa.

8. Garnish with fresh cilantro and enjoy.

Tofu Stir-Fry with Brown Rice (Vegan)

Ingredients:

- 1 block of firm tofu, drained and cubed
- Assorted stir-fry vegetables (such as bell peppers, broccoli, snap peas, and carrots)
- 2 tablespoons low-sodium soy sauce or tamari (gluten-free option)
- 1 tablespoon sesame oil
- 2 cloves garlic, minced
- 1 teaspoon grated fresh ginger
- Crushed red pepper flakes (optional)
- Cooked brown rice for serving

Preparation:

1. Heat the sesame oil in a big skillet or wok over medium-high heat.

2. Include the optional red pepper flakes, grated ginger, and chopped garlic. Stir-fry until aromatic, about 30 seconds.

3. Add the cubed tofu to the skillet and stir-fry until lightly browned on all sides.

4. Add the stir-fry vegetables and cook until they are tender-crisp, about 4-5 minutes.

5. Stir in the low-sodium soy sauce or tamari, making sure the tofu and vegetables are coated evenly.

6. Cook everything through for a further two to three minutes.

7. Serve the tofu stir-fry over cooked brown rice.

Greek Salad with Grilled Chicken (Non-Vegetarian)

Ingredients:
- 4 cups mixed salad greens
- 1 cup cherry tomatoes, halved
- 1/2 cup sliced cucumber
- 1/4 cup sliced red onion
- 1/2 cup Kalamata olives
- 1/2 cup crumbled feta cheese
- 2 grilled chicken breasts, sliced
- Juice of 1 lemon
- 2 tablespoons extra virgin olive oil
- Salt and pepper to taste

Preparation:

1. In a large salad bowl, combine the salad greens, cherry tomatoes, cucumber, red onion, Kalamata olives, and crumbled feta cheese.
2. Add the grilled chicken slices to the salad.
3. In a small bowl, whisk together the lemon juice and olive oil. Season with salt and pepper.
4. Drizzle the dressing over the salad and toss gently to combine.
5. Serve immediately.

Lentil Soup with Whole Grain Bread (Vegetarian/Vegan)

Ingredients:

- One cup of washed and drained dried lentils, either brown or green
- 1 onion, diced
- 2 carrots, diced
- 2 celery stalks, diced
- 3 cloves garlic, minced
- 1 can diced tomatoes
- 4 cups vegetable broth
- 1 teaspoon ground cumin
- 1 teaspoon ground coriander
- 1/2 teaspoon turmeric
- Salt and pepper to taste
- Fresh parsley or cilantro for garnish
- Whole grain bread for serving

Preparation:
1. Heat a small amount of oil in a big pot over medium heat.
2. Add the diced onion, carrots, celery, and garlic. The vegetables should soften after around five minutes of sautéing.
3. Add the lentils, diced tomatoes (with their juice), vegetable broth, cumin, coriander, turmeric, salt, and pepper to the pot. Stir well to combine.
4. Bring the soup to a boil, then reduce the heat to low and simmer for about 30-40 minutes, or until the lentils are tender.
5. If necessary, taste and adjust the seasoning.
6. Ladle the lentil soup into bowls and garnish with fresh parsley or cilantro.
7. Serve with whole grain bread on the side.

These lunch recipes are designed to provide a balance of protein, healthy fats, and low glycemic index carbs, which are beneficial for individuals with PCOS.

The recipes should provide you with a variety of options that are quick, easy, and suitable for individuals with PCOS. They emphasize the use of whole grains, lean proteins, and healthy fats while accommodating vegetarian and vegan diets. Enjoy your delicious and nutritious lunches.

CHAPTER SIX

Dinner Recipes

Here are flavorful and satisfying dinner recipes suitable for individuals with PCOS, emphasizing lean proteins, vegetables, and healthy fats, while being gluten-free and dairy-free:

Grilled Lemon Herb Chicken with Roasted Vegetables

Ingredients:
- 4 boneless, skinless chicken breasts
- 2 tablespoons olive oil
- Juice of 1 lemon
- 2 cloves garlic, minced
- 1 teaspoon dried thyme
- 1 teaspoon dried rosemary
- Salt and pepper to taste
- Assorted vegetables (such as bell peppers, zucchini, and cherry tomatoes), chopped

Method:
1. In a bowl, mix olive oil, lemon juice, minced garlic, dried thyme, dried rosemary, salt, and pepper.
2. Marinate the chicken breasts in the mixture for 30 minutes.
3. Preheat grill to medium-high heat.

4. Grill the chicken breasts for 6-8 minutes per side, or until cooked through.

5. While the chicken is grilling, toss the chopped vegetables with olive oil, salt, and pepper. Roast in the oven at 400°F (200°C) for 20-25 minutes, or until tender.

6. Serve the grilled chicken alongside the roasted vegetables.

Baked Salmon with Asparagus and Lemon

Ingredients:
- 4 salmon fillets
- 1 bunch asparagus, trimmed
- 2 tablespoons olive oil
- Juice of 1 lemon
- Salt and pepper to taste

Method:
1. Preheat the oven to 375°F (190°C).

2. Place salmon fillets and asparagus on a baking sheet lined with parchment paper.

3. Drizzle olive oil and lemon juice over the salmon and asparagus. Season with salt and pepper.

4. Bake the salmon for 12 to 15 minutes, or until it is cooked through and flake readily when tested with a fork.

5. Serve the baked salmon and asparagus hot.

Turkey and Vegetable Stir-Fry

Ingredients:
- 1 lb (450g) lean ground turkey

- 2 tablespoons coconut aminos (gluten-free soy sauce alternative)
- 2 cloves garlic, minced
- 1 teaspoon grated ginger
- Assorted vegetables (such as bell peppers, broccoli, carrots), sliced
- 2 tablespoons coconut oil
- Salt and pepper to taste
- Ready-to-eat cooked quinoa or cauliflower rice

Method:
1. In a skillet, heat coconut oil over medium heat. Add minced garlic and grated ginger, sauté until fragrant.
2. Add ground turkey to the skillet, breaking it up with a spatula. Cook until browned.
3. Stir in assorted vegetables and coconut aminos. Cook until the vegetables are tender.
4. To taste, add salt and pepper for seasoning.
5. Serve the turkey and vegetable stir-fry over cooked quinoa or cauliflower rice.

Lemon Garlic Shrimp with Zucchini Noodles

Ingredients:
- 1 lb (450g) shrimp, peeled and deveined
- 3-4 medium zucchini, spiralized into noodles
- 2 tablespoons olive oil
- Juice of 1 lemon
- 3 cloves garlic, minced
- Salt and pepper to taste

- Chopped fresh parsley, for garnish

Method:
1. Heat olive oil in a skillet over medium heat. When aromatic, add the minced garlic and simmer.
2. When the shrimp are pink and opaque, add them to the skillet and simmer.
3. Stir in zucchini noodles and lemon juice. Cook until the noodles are tender.
4. To taste, add salt and pepper for seasoning.
5. Before serving, garnish with freshly cut parsley.

Beef and Broccoli Stir-Fry

Ingredients:
- 1 lb (450g) flank steak, thinly sliced
- 2 tablespoons coconut aminos
- 2 cloves garlic, minced
- 1 teaspoon grated ginger
- 1 tablespoon coconut oil
- 4 cups broccoli florets
- Salt and pepper to taste
- Cooked rice or cauliflower rice, for serving

Method:
1. In a bowl, marinate sliced flank steak with coconut aminos, minced garlic, and grated ginger for 15-30 minutes.
2. In a skillet over medium heat, preheat the coconut oil. Cook the marinated steak until it turns golden brown.

3. Add broccoli florets to the skillet and stir-fry until tender-crisp.

4. Add pepper and salt to taste.

5. Serve the beef and broccoli stir-fry over cooked rice or cauliflower rice.

Stuffed Bell Peppers with Ground Turkey

Ingredients:
- 4 bell peppers, cut in half, and seeds taken out
- 1 lb (450g) lean ground turkey
- 1 onion, diced
- 2 cloves garlic, minced
- 1 can diced tomatoes, drained
- 1 teaspoon Italian seasoning
- Salt and pepper to taste
- Chopped fresh parsley, for garnish

Method:
1. Preheat the oven to 375°F (190°C).

2. In a skillet, cook ground turkey, diced onion, and minced garlic until turkey is browned and onions are softened.

3. Stir in diced tomatoes and Italian seasoning. Cook for an additional 5 minutes.

4. To taste, add salt and pepper for seasoning.

5. Fill each bell pepper half with the turkey mixture.

6. Place stuffed bell peppers in a baking dish and cover with foil. Bake peppers for 25 to 30 minutes, or until soft.

7. Garnish with chopped fresh parsley before serving.

Mediterranean Grilled Veggie Platter

Ingredients:
- Various veggies (including cherry tomatoes, bell peppers, zucchini, and eggplant)
- 2 tablespoons olive oil
- 2 cloves garlic, minced
- Juice of 1 lemon
- Salt and pepper to taste
- Fresh herbs for garnish (parsley, basil, etc.)

Method:
1. Preheat the grill to medium-high heat.
2. In a bowl, toss assorted vegetables with olive oil, minced garlic, lemon juice, salt, and pepper.
3. Grill the vegetables until tender and lightly charred, about 5-7 minutes per side.
4. Arrange grilled vegetables on a platter and garnish with fresh herbs.
5. Serve the Mediterranean grilled veggie platter with a side of hummus or quinoa.

Thai Coconut Curry with Chicken and Vegetables

Ingredients:
- One pound (450 grams) of skinless, boneless chicken breasts, sliced into little pieces
- 1 tablespoon coconut oil
- 1 onion, diced
- 2 cloves garlic, minced
- 1 tablespoon grated ginger
- 2 tablespoons Thai red curry paste

- One 13.5-ounce can of full-fat coconut milk
- Two cups of mixed veggies, including carrots, broccoli, and bell peppers
- 1 tablespoon coconut aminos
- Salt and pepper to taste
- Fresh cilantro, for garnish
- Cooked rice or cauliflower rice, for serving

Method:
1. Heat the coconut oil in a big skillet over medium heat. Add diced onion, minced garlic, and grated ginger. Sauté until fragrant.
2. Add chicken pieces to the skillet and cook until browned on all sides.
3. Stir in Thai red curry paste and cook for 1-2 minutes.
4. Pour in coconut milk and coconut aminos. Bring to a simmer.
5. Add assorted vegetables to the skillet and cook until tender.
6. To taste, add salt and pepper for seasoning.
7. Serve the Thai coconut curry over cooked rice or cauliflower rice. Garnish with fresh cilantro before serving.

Mediterranean Grilled Chicken Salad

Ingredients:
- 1 lb (450g) boneless, skinless chicken breasts
- 2 tablespoons olive oil
- Juice of 1 lemon
- 2 cloves garlic, minced

- 1 teaspoon dried oregano
- Salt and pepper to taste
- Mixed salad greens
- a variety of veggies (including red onion, cucumber, and cherry tomatoes)
- Kalamata olives, sliced
- Dairy-free feta cheese, crumbled (optional)
- Balsamic vinaigrette dressing (gluten-free and dairy-free), for serving

Method:
1. In a bowl, whisk together olive oil, lemon juice, minced garlic, dried oregano, salt, and pepper.
2. Marinate chicken breasts in the mixture for 30 minutes.
3. Preheat grill to medium-high heat.
4. Grill the chicken breasts for 6-8 minutes per side, or until cooked through.
5. Before slicing, let the chicken a few minutes to rest.
6. Arrange mixed salad greens, assorted vegetables, and sliced Kalamata olives on plates.
7. Top with sliced grilled chicken.
8. Sprinkle dairy-free feta cheese (if using) over the salad.
9. Drizzle with balsamic vinaigrette dressing before serving.

Teriyaki Glazed Salmon with Stir-Fried Vegetables

Ingredients:

- 4 salmon fillets
- 1/4 cup coconut aminos or gluten-free soy sauce
- 2 tablespoons honey or maple syrup
- 1 tablespoon rice vinegar
- 2 cloves garlic, minced
- 1 teaspoon grated ginger
- 1 tablespoon sesame oil
- Assorted vegetables (such as bell peppers, snap peas, carrots)
- Cooked rice or cauliflower rice, for serving

Method:
1. In a bowl, whisk together gluten-free soy sauce, honey or maple syrup, rice vinegar, minced garlic, and grated ginger to make the teriyaki glaze.
2. In a skillet over medium heat, warm the sesame oil. Add assorted vegetables and stir-fry until tender-crisp.
3. Remove vegetables from the skillet and set aside.
4. Add salmon fillets to the skillet and cook for 3-4 minutes per side.
5. Pour the teriyaki glaze over the salmon and cook for an additional 1-2 minutes, until the glaze thickens.
6. Serve the teriyaki glazed salmon with stir-fried vegetables and cooked rice or cauliflower rice.

Zucchini Noodles with Pesto Shrimp

Ingredients:
- 1 lb (450g) shrimp, peeled and deveined

- 2 tablespoons olive oil
- 2 cloves garlic, minced
- 3 cups zucchini noodles (zoodles)
- 1/2 cup dairy-free pesto sauce
- Salt and pepper to taste
- Cherry tomatoes, halved, for garnish
- Fresh basil leaves, for garnish

Method:
1. Heat olive oil in a skillet over medium heat. When aromatic, add the minced garlic and simmer.
2. When the shrimp are pink and opaque, add them to the skillet and simmer.
3. Stir in zucchini noodles and cook until tender.
4. Add dairy-free pesto sauce to the skillet and toss until well combined.
5. Add pepper and salt to taste.
6. Garnish with halved cherry tomatoes and fresh basil leaves before serving.

Taco Stuffed Sweet Potatoes

Ingredients:
- 4 medium sweet potatoes
- One pound (450g) of lean ground chicken or turkey
- 1 tablespoon olive oil
- 1 onion, diced
- 2 cloves garlic, minced
- 1 tablespoon chili powder
- 1 teaspoon ground cumin
- 1/2 teaspoon paprika

- Salt and pepper to taste
- Avocado slices, for topping
- Salsa, for topping
- Fresh cilantro, for garnish

Method:
1. Preheat the oven to 400°F (200°C).
2. Prick sweet potatoes with a fork and place them on a baking sheet. Bake until soft, 45 to 50 minutes.
3. While the sweet potatoes are baking, heat olive oil in a skillet over medium heat. Saute the minced garlic and diced onion until they become tender.
4. Add ground turkey or chicken to the skillet and cook until browned.
5. Stir in chili powder, ground cumin, paprika, salt, and pepper. Cook for an additional 2-3 minutes.
6. Once the sweet potatoes are cooked, slice them open and fluff the insides with a fork.
7. Spoon the taco meat mixture over the sweet potatoes.
8. Top with avocado slices, salsa, and fresh cilantro before serving.

These dinner recipes offer a variety of flavorful and satisfying options for individuals with PCOS, focusing on lean proteins, vegetables, and healthy fats while being gluten-free and dairy-free. Enjoy these nutritious meals as part of a balanced diet.

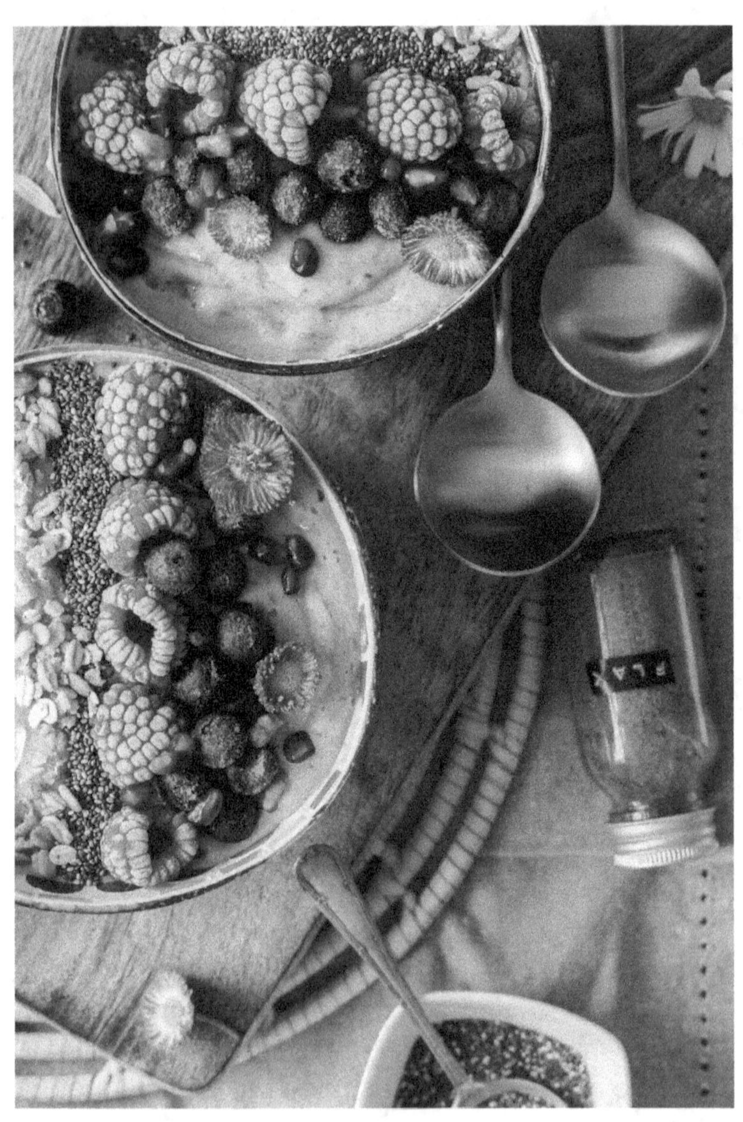

CHAPTER SEVEN

Snacks and Desserts

Here are snack and dessert recipes that are PCOS-friendly, delicious, and emphasize the use of whole foods and natural sweeteners. I've also included options for gluten-free and dairy-free diets:

Energy Balls

Ingredients:
- One cup of almonds, or any other type of nuts
- 1 cup pitted dates
- 2 tablespoons unsweetened cocoa powder (or cacao powder)
- 1 tablespoon of nut butter, such as almond butter
- 1 tablespoon chia seeds (optional)
- 1 teaspoon vanilla extract
- Pinch of salt

Instructions:
- Place all ingredients in a food processor and blend until well combined and sticky.
- Roll the mixture into small balls.
- To firm up, refrigerate for a minimum of half an hour.

Chia Pudding

Ingredients:
- 1/4 cup chia seeds

-One cup of unsweetened almond milk (or your preferred dairy-free milk)
- 1 tablespoon pure maple syrup (or any natural sweetener)
- 1/2 teaspoon vanilla extract
- Fresh berries for topping

Instructions:
- In a jar or bowl, mix together chia seeds, almond milk, maple syrup, and vanilla extract.
- After giving it a good stir, wait five minutes.
- Stir again to break up any clumps, then refrigerate overnight or for at least 4 hours.
- Top with fresh berries before serving.

Baked Apple Chips

Ingredients:
- 2 apples (any variety)
- Cinnamon powder

Instructions:
- Preheat your oven to 200°C (400°F).
- Using a sharp knife or mandoline, finely slice the apples.
- Place the apple slices on a baking sheet lined with parchment paper.
- Dredge the apple slices in cinnamon powder.
- Bake for about 1 hour or until the chips are crispy. Let them cool completely before enjoying.

Avocado Chocolate Pudding

Ingredients:
- 2 ripe avocados
- 1/4 cup unsweetened cocoa powder
- 1/4 cup pure maple syrup (or any natural sweetener)
- 1/4 cup unsweetened almond milk (or any dairy-free milk of your choice)
- 1 teaspoon vanilla extract
- Pinch of salt

Instructions:
- Scoop the avocado flesh into a blender or food processor.
- Add cocoa powder, maple syrup, almond milk, vanilla extract, and salt.
- Blend until smooth and creamy.
- Transfer to serving dishes and refrigerate for at least 30 minutes before serving.

Roasted Chickpeas

Ingredients:
- 1 can chickpeas, drained and rinsed
- 1 tablespoon olive oil
- 1 teaspoon ground cumin
- 1/2 teaspoon smoked paprika
- 1/2 teaspoon garlic powder
- Salt and pepper to taste

Instructions:
- Preheat your oven to 200°C (400°F).

- Pat dry the chickpeas with a clean kitchen towel.
- Chickpeas should be combined with olive oil, salt, pepper, cumin, smoked paprika, and garlic powder in a bowl.
- Arrange the chickpeas on a baking sheet in a single layer.
- Roast the chickpeas for 25 to 30 minutes, shaking the pan from time to time, or until they become crispy.
- Let them cool before enjoying.

Greek Yogurt Parfait (dairy-free option)

Ingredients:
- One cup of dairy-free yogurt, like almond or coconut yogurt
- 1/4 cup fresh berries
- 1 tablespoon chopped nuts (such as almonds or walnuts)
- 1 tablespoon unsweetened shredded coconut
- One teaspoon of pure maple syrup or honey (optional)

Instructions:
- In a glass or jar, layer the dairy-free yogurt, fresh berries, chopped nuts, and shredded coconut.
- If desired, drizzle with maple syrup or honey.
- Continue layering until all of the ingredients have been utilized.
- Eat right away or store in the fridge until you're ready.

Banana Ice Cream

Ingredients:
- 2 ripe bananas, peeled and sliced
- 1 tablespoon of nut butter, such as almond butter
- 1/2 teaspoon vanilla extract
- Optional toppings: chopped nuts, dark chocolate chips, coconut flakes

Instructions:
- Place the sliced bananas in a ziplock bag and freeze for at least 2 hours or until solid.
- In a blender or food processor, add the frozen bananas, almond butter, and vanilla extract.
- Scrape down the sides as necessary, and blend until creamy and smooth.
- Serve immediately, topped with your favorite toppings if desired.

No-Bake Almond Butter Bars (gluten-free)

Ingredients:
- 1 cup almond butter
- 1/4 cup pure maple syrup (or any natural sweetener)
- 1/4 cup coconut oil, melted
- 1/2 teaspoon vanilla extract
- 2 cups gluten-free rolled oats
- 1/4 cup unsweetened shredded coconut
- 1/4 cup dark chocolate chips (optional)

Instructions:

-Almond butter, maple syrup, melted coconut oil, and vanilla extract should all be combined in a large mixing basin.

- Stir in the rolled oats, shredded coconut, and dark chocolate chips (if using), until well combined.

- Press the mixture into a lined baking dish or pan.

- Place in the refrigerator until solid, at least 2 hours.

- Cut into bars and enjoy!

Berry Smoothie Bowl

Ingredients:

- 1 cup frozen mixed berries
- 1 ripe banana
- 1/2 cup unsweetened almond milk (or any dairy-free milk of your choice)
- 1 tablespoon chia seeds
- Toppings: fresh berries, sliced almonds, coconut flakes, granola

Instructions:

- In a blender, combine frozen berries, banana, almond milk, and chia seeds.

- Blend until smooth and creamy.

- Pour the smoothie into a bowl and top with fresh berries, sliced almonds, coconut flakes, and granola.

- Enjoy with a spoon!

Quinoa Chocolate Chip Cookies (gluten-free, dairy-free)

Ingredients:
- 1 cup cooked quinoa, cooled
- 1 cup gluten-free oat flour
- 1/2 cup almond flour
- 1/4 cup coconut sugar
- 1/4 cup pure maple syrup (or any natural sweetener)
- 1/4 cup coconut oil, melted
- 1 teaspoon vanilla extract
- 1/2 teaspoon baking powder
- 1/4 teaspoon salt
- 1/2 cup dark chocolate chips

Instructions:
- Preheat your oven to 180°C (350°F) and line a baking sheet with parchment paper.
- In a large mixing bowl, combine cooked quinoa, oat flour, almond flour, coconut sugar, maple syrup, coconut oil, vanilla extract, baking powder, and salt. Mix well.
- Fold in the dark chocolate chips.
- Drop dough onto the baking sheet that has been prepared by spoonfuls.
- Bake for twelve to fifteen minutes, or until very lightly browned.
- After a few minutes of cooling on the baking sheet, move the cookies to a wire rack to finish cooling.

These snack and dessert recipes should provide you with a variety of options that are PCOS-friendly, delicious, and incorporate whole foods and natural sweeteners. They also include options for gluten-free and dairy-free diets. Enjoy these treats while nourishing your body.

CHAPTER EIGHT

Meal Planning and Preparation Tips

Strategies for meal planning

To support a PCOS-friendly diet, meal planning and preparation should focus on balancing protein, non-starchy vegetables, and whole grains, while minimizing refined carbohydrates and added sugars. Here are some strategies for meal planning and preparation to support a PCOS-friendly diet:

1. Balanced Meals: When planning meals, aim to make 1/4 of the plate protein, 1/2 of the plate non-starchy vegetables, and 1/4 of the plate starchy vegetables or whole grains. This helps in balancing blood sugar levels and managing insulin resistance.

2. Lean Proteins: Include lean proteins such as grilled chicken, turkey breast, fish, lentils, and beans in your meals. These proteins help in managing blood sugar levels and keeping you full for longer.

3. Non-Starchy Vegetables: Prioritize non-starchy vegetables like leafy greens, broccoli, cauliflower,

and bell peppers. These vegetables are rich in fiber and nutrients, and they have a lower impact on blood sugar levels.

4. Whole Grains: Choose whole grains such as quinoa, brown rice, and oats over refined grains. Whole grains provide fiber and are digested more slowly, which can help with blood sugar control.

5. Healthy Fats: Include fats that are good for you, such as those found in olive oil, avocados, nuts, and seeds. Healthy fats are important for hormone production and can help with managing inflammation, which is beneficial for individuals with PCOS.

6. Meal Timing: Eating three full meals and one snack, and spacing them out four to six hours apart, is a good strategy to follow for PCOS. This allows insulin levels to come into balance and supports blood sugar regulation.

7. Meal Prep: Consider preparing some meal components in advance, such as cooking a batch of whole grains, roasting vegetables, or grilling a few servings of lean protein. This can make it easier to assemble balanced meals throughout the week, especially during busy days.

By following these strategies, individuals with PCOS can create well-balanced meals that support blood sugar regulation, hormone balance, and overall health.

Tips on how to control your appetite and eat a balanced diet

Managing food cravings and maintaining a balanced diet can be important for individuals with PCOS. Here are some tips to help:

1. Eat Regular Meals: Stick to a regular eating schedule with balanced meals throughout the day. This can help stabilize blood sugar levels and prevent extreme hunger or cravings.

2. Include Protein and Healthy Fats: Incorporate protein-rich foods such as lean meats, fish, eggs, legumes, and tofu in your meals. Also, include healthy fats like avocados, nuts, seeds, and olive oil. Protein and healthy fats can help you feel satisfied and reduce cravings.

3. Choose Complex Carbohydrates: Opt for complex carbohydrates that have a lower glycemic index, such as whole grains, sweet potatoes, quinoa, and legumes. These carbs are digested more slowly, providing sustained energy and helping to stabilize blood sugar levels.

4. Fiber-Rich Foods: Include plenty of fiber in your diet from fruits, vegetables, whole grains, and legumes. Fiber helps regulate blood sugar levels and promotes a feeling of fullness, reducing cravings.

5. Keep Yourself Hydrated: Occasionally, thirst might be confused with hunger or desires. Stay hydrated by drinking enough water throughout the day to help curb unnecessary food cravings.

6. Mindful Eating: Practice mindful eating by paying attention to your body's hunger and fullness cues. Take the time to savor and enjoy your meals, eating slowly and without distractions. This can help you better tune in to your body's needs and prevent overeating or emotional eating.

7. Plan and Prepare Meals: Plan your meals and snacks in advance to avoid impulsive food choices or relying on unhealthy options. Prepare meals at home using whole and natural ingredients whenever possible. This gives you more control over the quality and nutritional content of your meals.

8. Handle Stress: Emotional eating and cravings can be brought on by stress. Find healthy ways to manage stress, such as practicing relaxation techniques, engaging in physical activity, getting enough sleep, or participating in activities you enjoy.

Always keep in mind that it's critical to strike a balance that suits your unique wants and requirements. Be patient with yourself and focus on nourishing your body with wholesome, nutrient-dense foods while allowing for occasional treats in moderation.

CHAPTER NINE

PCOS-friendly ingredient substitutions

PCOS, also known as polycystic ovarian syndrome, is a hormonal condition affecting individuals, mostly women who are fertile. Dietary modifications are often recommended as part of managing PCOS symptoms, including insulin resistance, weight gain, and hormonal imbalances. Making PCOS-friendly ingredient substitutions can help individuals maintain a balanced diet and support their overall health. Here's a comprehensive guide to PCOS-friendly ingredient substitutions:

1.Carbohydrates

- Substitute refined grains with whole grains: Choose whole grains like brown rice, quinoa, buckwheat, and oats instead of white rice, white bread, and pasta. Whole grains have a lower glycemic index and provide more fiber, which helps regulate blood sugar levels.

- Replace sugary snacks with low-glycemic alternatives: Opt for snacks like nuts, seeds, and fresh fruits, which have a lower impact on blood sugar levels compared to sugary treats and desserts.

2. **Dairy**

- Use dairy-free alternatives: Replace cow's milk with plant-based milk alternatives like almond milk, coconut milk, soy milk, or oat milk. These alternatives are lower in saturated fats and may be better tolerated by individuals with lactose intolerance or dairy sensitivities.

- Choose dairy-free yogurt and cheese: Look for dairy-free yogurt made from coconut, almond, soy, or oat milk. Dairy-free cheese alternatives are also available and can be used in cooking and as toppings.

3. **Proteins**

- Select lean protein sources: Include lean protein sources such as skinless poultry, fish, tofu, tempeh, legumes, and lentils in your diet. These proteins are lower in saturated fats and can help support muscle maintenance and repair.

- Opt for plant-based proteins: Incorporate plant-based protein sources like beans, lentils, chickpeas, and quinoa to increase fiber intake and promote satiety.

4. **Fats**

- Choose healthy fats: Replace saturated and trans fats with healthier options like olive oil, avocado oil, coconut oil, nuts, seeds, and avocados. These fats support heart health and may help reduce inflammation associated with PCOS.

- Limit processed and fried foods: Minimize consumption of processed foods, fried foods, and hydrogenated oils, which can contribute to inflammation and insulin resistance.

5. Sweeteners

- Use natural sweeteners sparingly: Instead of refined sugars, opt for natural sweeteners like honey, maple syrup, stevia, or monk fruit sweetener in moderation. Pay attention to portion sizes to prevent consuming too much sugar.

6. Sodium

- Reduce sodium intake: Limit the use of table salt and processed foods high in sodium. Use herbs, spices, and citrus juices to enhance flavor without relying on salt.

7. Fiber

- Increase fiber intake: Incorporate high-fiber foods such as fruits, vegetables, whole grains, legumes, nuts, and seeds into your diet. Fiber helps regulate blood sugar levels, promote digestive health, and support weight management.

8. Alcohol and Caffeine

- Moderate alcohol and caffeine consumption: Limit alcohol and caffeine intake, as excessive consumption may disrupt hormone balance and exacerbate PCOS symptoms. Opt for herbal teas and water as alternative beverages.

9. **Processed Foods**

- Minimize processed foods: Reduce consumption of processed and packaged foods containing artificial additives, preservatives, and refined ingredients. Choose whole, minimally processed foods whenever possible to support overall health and well-being.

By incorporating these PCOS-friendly ingredient substitutions into your diet, you can make healthier choices that may help manage symptoms and support your overall health and well-being. It's important to consult with a healthcare professional or registered dietitian for personalized dietary recommendations tailored to your individual needs and preferences.

Meal planning templates and grocery lists

Meal planning templates and grocery lists are essential tools for organizing meals, managing budgets, and maintaining a balanced diet. They help streamline the meal preparation process, reduce food waste, and ensure that you have the necessary ingredients on hand to create nutritious meals throughout the week. Here's a comprehensive guide to meal planning templates and grocery lists:

Meal Planning Templates

1. Weekly Meal Planner:

- A weekly meal planner allows you to map out your meals for the entire week, including breakfast, lunch, dinner, and snacks.

- Divide each day into sections for meal categories and jot down meal ideas or specific recipes you plan to prepare.

- Consider factors like dietary preferences, nutritional balance, and convenience when selecting meals for each day.

2. Monthly Meal Calendar:

- A monthly meal calendar provides a broader overview of your meal plan for the entire month.

- It allows for long-term planning, helping you incorporate seasonal ingredients, special occasions, and recurring meal themes into your schedule.

3. Batch Cooking Plan:

- Batch cooking involves preparing large quantities of meals in advance and portioning them out for future consumption.

- Create a batch cooking plan to schedule specific days for meal prep and designate which meals you'll prepare in bulk.

4. Theme Nights:

- Theme nights add variety to your meal plan and make meal planning more fun and engaging.

- Choose themes such as Meatless Mondays, Taco Tuesdays, Stir-Fry Fridays, or Soup Sundays to guide your meal selection for each day of the week.

5. Leftovers Utilization Plan:

- Incorporate leftover ingredients from previous meals into your meal plan to minimize food waste.

- Plan meals that use similar ingredients to maximize freshness and reduce the need for additional grocery shopping.

Grocery Lists

1. Categorized Lists:

- Organize your grocery list into categories such as produce, dairy, protein, grains, pantry staples, and miscellaneous items.

- Grouping similar items together makes shopping more efficient and helps prevent overlooking essential ingredients.

2. Meal-Specific Lists:

- Create separate grocery lists for each meal or recipe to ensure you have all the necessary ingredients on hand.

- Check your meal planning templates to identify which ingredients you'll need for each recipe and add them to the corresponding grocery list.

3. Quantity and Measurement:

- Specify quantities and measurements for each item on your grocery list to prevent overbuying or underbuying.

- Estimate the amount of ingredients you'll need based on the number of servings and adjust quantities accordingly.

4. Seasonal and Sale Items:
   - Take advantage of seasonal produce and sales by incorporating them into your grocery list.
   - Plan your meals around seasonal ingredients to save money and enjoy fresh, flavorful dishes.

5. Healthy Options:
   - Prioritize nutrient-dense foods and whole ingredients when creating your grocery list.
   - Include a variety of fruits, vegetables, lean proteins, whole grains, and healthy fats to support a balanced diet.

6. Staple Items:
   - Ensure your pantry is stocked with staple items such as rice, pasta, canned goods, spices, and condiments.
   - Regularly check your pantry inventory and add any depleted items to your grocery list.

7. Optional Items:
   - Leave space on your grocery list for optional items or impulse purchases.
   - Exercise mindfulness and avoid unnecessary purchases by sticking to your predetermined list and budget.

By utilizing meal planning templates and grocery lists, you can streamline your meal preparation process, make healthier food choices, and stay organized throughout the week. Whether you prefer digital or physical formats, finding a system that works for you will help simplify meal planning and grocery shopping while promoting a balanced and sustainable approach to eating.

CHAPTER TEN

Additional Resources

10 Weeks Grocery List

Here's a sample grocery list for a PCOS-friendly diet, spread over a 52-week period. This list includes a variety of nutrient-dense foods that can support a balanced diet for individuals with PCOS. You can adjust the quantities based on your needs and preferences:

Week 1:

- Chicken breasts
- Salmon fillets
- Ground turkey
- Eggs
- Greek yogurt (dairy-free if needed)
- Almond milk (unsweetened)
- Spinach
- Broccoli
- Bell peppers
- Tomatoes
- Sweet potatoes
- Quinoa
- Brown rice
- Oats (gluten-free if needed)
- Chia seeds
- Almonds

- Walnuts
- Avocados
- Berries
- Apples
- Lemons
- Olive oil
- Coconut oil
- Spices and herbs (such cinnamon, turmeric, ginger, and garlic)

Week 2:

- Lean beef
- Shrimp
- Tofu
- Cottage cheese (dairy-free if needed)
- Unsweetened almond butter
- Cucumber
- Carrots
- Zucchini
- Cauliflower
- Green beans
- Onions
- Quinoa pasta (gluten-free)
- Lentils
- Flaxseeds
- Pumpkin seeds
- Pecans
- Oranges
- Grapes
- Strawberries
- Limes

- Balsamic vinegar
- Tamari sauce (gluten-free soy sauce)

Week 3:

- Pork tenderloin
- White fish (such as cod or tilapia)
- Canned tuna (in water)
- Cashew milk (unsweetened)
- Kale
- Brussels sprouts
- Asparagus
- Mushrooms
- Eggplant
- Brown rice pasta (gluten-free)
- Black beans
- Hemp seeds
- Brazil nuts
- Pears
- Blueberries
- Raspberries
- Grapefruit
- Apple cider vinegar
- Dijon mustard

Week 4:

- Ground chicken
- Turkey bacon
- Non-dairy cheese
- Celery
- Beets
- Cabbage

- Butternut squash
- Gluten-free bread
- Chickpeas
- Sesame seeds
- Cashews
- Kiwi
- Mango
- Pineapple
- Papaya
- Coconut milk (unsweetened)
- Coconut flour
- Almond flour
- Stevia (natural sweetener)
- Cacao powder

Week 5:

- Chicken thighs
- Sardines (canned in water)
- Almond milk yogurt (unsweetened)
- Baby spinach
- Green peas
- Bell peppers
- Cilantro
- Butternut squash
- Buckwheat noodles (gluten-free)
- Black rice
- Quinoa flakes
- Pistachios
- Macadamia nuts
- Bananas
- Blackberries

- Cherries
- Dates
- Coconut water
- Nutritional yeast

Week 6:

- Ground lamb
- Cod fillets
- Full-fat coconut milk
- Romaine lettuce
- Kale
- Radishes
- Jicama
- Spaghetti squash
- Black lentils
- Sunflower seeds
- Hazelnuts
- Apricots
- Peaches
- Plums
- Watermelon
- Dried unsweetened coconut flakes
- Xylitol (natural sweetener)
- Turmeric powder

Week 7:

- Grass-fed beef
- Halibut fillets
- Cashew milk yogurt (unsweetened)
- Arugula
- Cabbage

- Swiss chard
- Egg noodles (gluten-free)
- Wild rice
- Amaranth
- Pomegranate seeds
- Brazil nuts
- Mangoes
- Papayas
- Pears
- Lemongrass
- Ghee (clarified butter)
- Green tea

Week 8:

- Turkey breasts
- Mackerel fillets
- Coconut milk yogurt (unsweetened)
- Baby kale
- Bok choy
- Radicchio
- Shirataki noodles
- Red lentils
- Poppy seeds
- Pine nuts
- Grapefruit
- Oranges
- Persimmons
- Prunes
- Sesame oil
- Apple cider vinegar

Week 9:

- Ground bison
- Rainbow trout fillets
- Rice milk (unsweetened)
- Watercress
- Endive
- Fennel
- Chickpea pasta (gluten-free)
- Pinto beans
- Pecans
- Kiwis
- Cranberries
- Guava
- Lychees
- Miso paste
- Tamari sauce (gluten-free soy sauce)

Week 10:

- Ground pork
- Tuna steaks
- Hemp milk (unsweetened)
- Dandelion greens
- Mustard greens
- Collard greens
- Kelp noodles
- Green lentils
- Sesame seeds
- Almonds
- Raspberries
- Gooseberries
- Nectarines

- Olives
- Apple sauce

Repeat these ten weeks for the remaining weeks of the year, and feel free to adjust the list based on your preferences and seasonal availability. Remember to prioritize nutrient-dense, whole foods, and vary your choices for a well-rounded diet.

Sample Meal Plan

Creating a 52-week sample meal plan for PCOS patients involves incorporating a variety of nutrient-dense foods, focusing on lean proteins, complex carbohydrates, healthy fats, and plenty of fruits and vegetables. Below is a general guideline for a weekly meal plan designed to support individuals with PCOS:

Week 1

Monday:

- Breakfast: Greek yogurt with berries and almonds
- Lunch: Quinoa salad with mixed greens, chickpeas, cucumber, and avocado
- Dinner is steamed broccoli, roasted sweet potatoes, and baked salmon.

Tuesday:

- Breakfast: Spinach and feta omelet with whole grain toast
- Lunch: Turkey and vegetable stir-fry with brown rice
- Dinner is a mixed green salad on the side and lentil soup.

Wednesday:

- Breakfast: Chia seed pudding with sliced bananas and walnuts
- Lunch: Grilled chicken salad with mixed vegetables and balsamic vinaigrette
- Dinner: Spaghetti squash with marinara sauce and lean ground turkey

Thursday:

- Breakfast: Smoothie with spinach, banana, almond milk, and protein powder
- Lunch: Quinoa and black bean stuffed bell peppers
- Dinner: Baked cod with quinoa pilaf and roasted asparagus

Friday:

- Breakfast consists of almond milk, mixed berries, chia seeds, and overnight oats.
- Lunch: Chickpea salad with cucumbers, tomatoes, and lemon-tahini dressing

- Supper is brown rice and broccoli with stir-fried tofu.

Saturday:

- Breakfast: Scrambled eggs with sautéed spinach and whole grain toast
- Lunch: Greek salad with grilled chicken and olives
- Dinner: Vegetable curry with cauliflower rice

Sunday:

- Breakfast: Oatmeal topped with sliced apples, cinnamon, and almonds
- Lunch: Lentil and vegetable soup with a side of quinoa salad
- Dinner: Grilled shrimp skewers with quinoa tabbouleh and roasted vegetables

Week 2-52:
- Follow a similar pattern, rotating through different proteins, grains, and vegetables to ensure variety and balanced nutrition.
- Incorporate seasonal produce and adapt recipes based on availability and preference.
- Experiment with different cooking methods and flavors to keep meals interesting and enjoyable.
- Observe serving sizes and pay attention to your body's signals of hunger and fullness.
- Stay hydrated throughout the day and consider incorporating herbal teas and infused water for added variety.

Customize the meal plan based on individual preferences, dietary restrictions, and nutritional needs. Consult with a healthcare professional or registered dietitian for personalized guidance and support in managing PCOS symptoms through nutrition and lifestyle modifications.

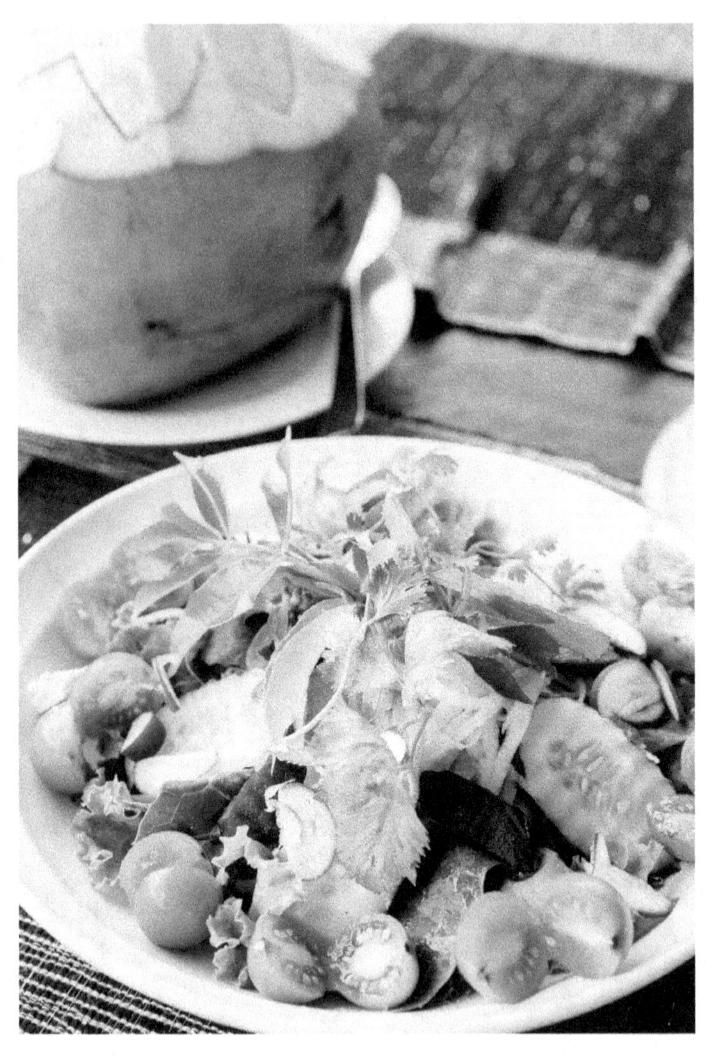

CONCLUSION

In closing, the journey through the pages of this book has been one of discovery, empowerment, and transformation in the realm of Polycystic Ovary Syndrome (PCOS) management. As we conclude this comprehensive guide, it's essential to reflect on the key takeaways and insights gained along the way.

Understanding PCOS: We embarked on this journey by delving into the intricate nature of PCOS, unraveling its multifaceted symptoms, underlying causes, and impact on women's health. Armed with knowledge, we empowered ourselves to recognize the signs, seek appropriate medical care, and embrace proactive strategies for managing PCOS effectively.

Importance of Diet and Lifestyle: Central to our exploration was the recognition of the pivotal role that diet and lifestyle play in mitigating PCOS symptoms and promoting overall well-being. Through the adoption of a balanced, nutrient-dense diet, rich in whole foods, lean proteins, fruits, vegetables, and healthy fats, we nourished our bodies and cultivated resilience against hormonal imbalances and metabolic disruptions.

Lifestyle Modifications: We embraced lifestyle modifications as powerful tools in our arsenal against PCOS, incorporating regular physical activity, stress management techniques, adequate sleep, and weight management strategies into our daily routines. By prioritizing self-care and mindfulness, we fostered a holistic approach to health that transcended mere symptom management to encompass the cultivation of vitality and vitality.

Empowerment through Knowledge: At the heart of our journey lies the recognition that knowledge is power. By equipping ourselves with evidence-based information, practical strategies, and empowering resources, we reclaimed agency over our health and embarked on a path of self-discovery, growth, and empowerment.

Celebrating Progress and Resilience: As we bid farewell to these pages, let us celebrate the progress made, the victories won, and the resilience forged in the face of adversity. Each step taken, each choice made, and each lesson learned has brought us closer to a place of healing, wholeness, and self-empowerment.

In conclusion, may this book serve as a beacon of hope, guidance, and inspiration to all those navigating the challenges of PCOS. May it embolden us to embrace our journeys with courage, compassion, and unwavering determination. And may it remind us that, through knowledge, empowerment, and community, we possess the strength to thrive, flourish, and shine brightly in the face of adversity.

As we turn the final page, let us carry forth the wisdom gained, the lessons learned, and the bonds forged, knowing that together, we stand strong, resilient, and empowered in the pursuit of health, happiness, and wholeness.

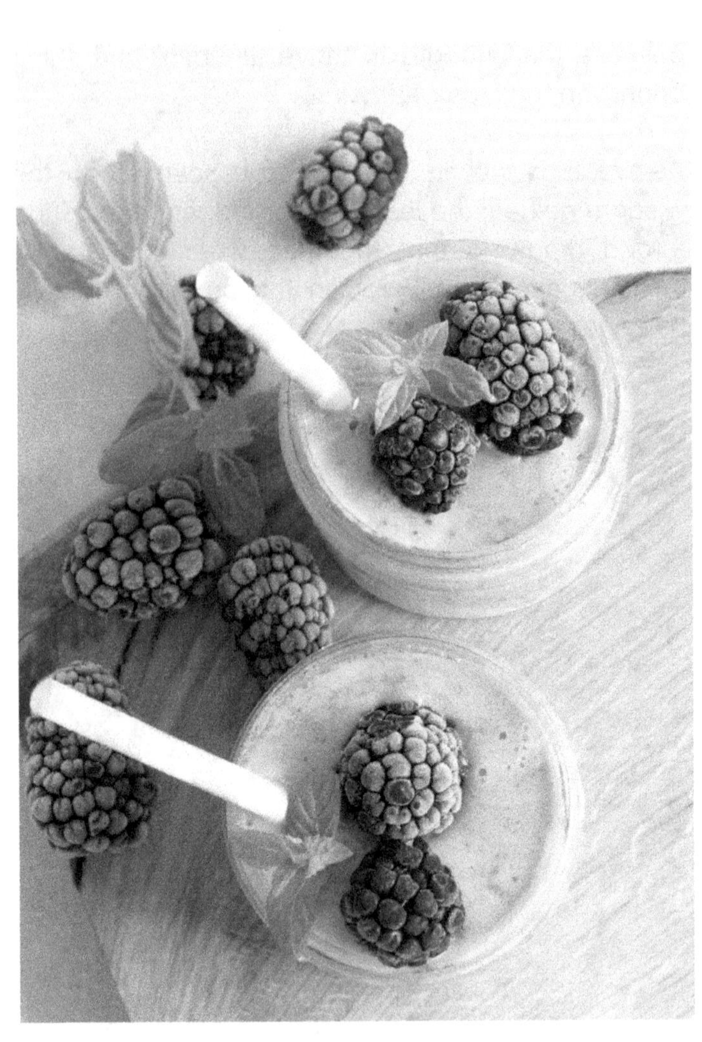

Appendix

Conversion Table

Here is a conversion table for common units of measurement used in the book:

Length:
- 1 inch (in) = 2.54 centimeters (cm)
- 1 foot (ft) = 30.48 centimeters (cm)
- 1 meter (m) = 3.281 feet (ft)

Weight:
- 1 ounce (oz) = 28.35 grams (g)
- 1 pound (lb) = 0.4536 kilograms (kg)
- 1 kilogram (kg) = 2.205 pounds (lb)

Volume:
- 1 teaspoon (tsp) = 5 milliliters (ml)
- 1 tablespoon (tbsp) = 15 milliliters (ml)
- 1 fluid ounce (fl oz) = 29.573 milliliters (ml)
- 1 cup = 236.59 milliliters (ml)
- 1 liter (l) = 33.814 fluid ounces (fl oz)

Temperature:
- Fahrenheit to Celsius: (°F - 32) × 5/9 = °C
- Celsius to Fahrenheit: (°C × 9/5) + 32 = °F

Time:
- 1 minute (min) = 60 seconds (s)
- 1 hour (hr) = 60 minutes (min)

- 1 day = 24 hours (hr)
- 1 week = 7 days
- 1 month ≈ 30.44 days
- 1 year ≈ 365.25 days

This conversion table helps readers understand and adapt measurements as needed while following recipes, guidelines, and recommendations provided in the book.

www.ingramcontent.com/pod-product-compliance
Lightning Source LLC
Chambersburg PA
CBHW070838250726
48662CB00003B/1282